LAST-MINUTE
OPTICS

A Concise Review of
Optics, Refraction, and Contact Lenses

THIRD
EDITION

LAST-MINUTE
OPTICS

A Concise Review of
Optics, Refraction, and Contact Lenses

David G. Hunter, MD, PhD
Ophthalmologist-in-Chief
Department of Ophthalmology
Boston Children's Hospital
Professor and Vice Chair of Ophthalmology
Harvard Medical School
Boston, Massachusetts
USA

Michael J. Wan, MD, FRCSC
Pediatric Ophthalmologist
Department of Ophthalmology and Vision Sciences
Sick Kids Hospital
Assistant Professor
University of Toronto
Toronto, Ontario
Canada

Constance E. West, MD
Retired Ophthalmologist
Ossipee, New Hampshire
USA

ELSEVIER

Elsevier

1600 John F. Kennedy Blvd.
Ste 1800
Philadelphia, PA 19103-2899

LAST-MINUTE OPTICS: A CONCISE REVIEW OF OPTICS,   ISBN: 978-0-443-12807-3
REFRACTION, AND CONTACT LENSES, THIRD EDITION

Notice

Practitioners and researchers must always rely on their own experience and knowledge in evaluating and using any information, methods, compounds, or experiments described herein. Because of rapid advances in the medical sciences, in particular, independent verification of diagnoses and drug dosages should be made. To the fullest extent of the law, no responsibility is assumed by Elsevier, authors, editors, or contributors for any injury and/or damage to persons or property as a matter of product liability, negligence or otherwise, or from any use or operation of any methods, products, instructions, or ideas contained in the material herein.

Previous editions copyrighted 2nd edition—2010 by Slack Incorporated,
1st edition—1996 by Slack Incorporated

Executive Content Strategist: Kayla Wolfe
Senior Content Development Specialist: Jinia Dasgupta
Publishing Services Manager: Shereen Jameel
Project Manager: Gayathri S.
Design Direction: Margaret M. Reid

Printed in India

Last digit is the print number: 9 8 7 6 5 4 3 2 1

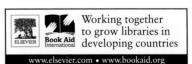

Working together
to grow libraries in
developing countries

www.elsevier.com • www.bookaid.org

This book is dedicated to Dr. David Guyton and to all the people who have supported us and inspired us to teach optics.

"Optics is hard."
"Optics is irrelevant."
"I hate optics."

These are the battle cries we have heard from our students over the years as they embark on yet another annual attempt to review optics (i.e., cram at the last minute). We like to think that the cries die down by the time we finish our lectures (hopefully due to enhanced understanding and not just sleep and surrender). We believe that this book captures our approach to our lectures on the subject, making optics accessible and understandable, clinically relevant, and maybe even (gasp) fun at times.

This is not a comprehensive treatise on optics. Our goal is to present the most relevant concepts of optics concisely, for those who have a limited amount of time to study. We use a question-and-answer format to help you identify weak areas while at the same time reviewing the key concepts to reinforce areas you already understand. While the laws of physics have not changed substantially since the last edition, clinical care has moved forward enough that it was time for another comprehensive revision. In creating this third edition, we spent considerable time reviewing and revising the entire text (while leaving the good stuff alone). We also added a third coauthor (M.J.W.) from Canada (an expert on the metric system and polite *humour*). We have significantly enhanced the illustrations and added a new feature called "Exam Pearls" in which we give our top exam tips on the highest-yield material.

The knowledge gained in reading this book is not just trivia that might help you pass an exam. It is real-life optics taken (for the most part) from our experience with real-life patients—an approach that we hope will make you a better doctor, empower you to enjoy your optics-related patient encounters, and perhaps even help you pass those pesky exams.

David G. Hunter, MD, PhD

Michael J. Wan, MD, FRCSC

Constance E. West, MD

CONTENTS

CHAPTER 1

Refraction and Reflection

1. What is the refractive index (n) and how is it calculated?

The refractive index (n) is a characteristic of a given optical medium related to how fast light passes through that material. It is calculated as the ratio of the speed of light in a vacuum to the speed of light in that material (Fig. 1.1).

$$n_{medium} = \frac{\text{speed of light in a vacuum}}{\text{speed of light in the medium}}$$

Fig. 1.1 Formula to calculate the refractive index of a given medium.

2. Can the refractive index ever be less than 1.000?

No!

According to some guy named Albert Einstein, nothing in the universe can travel faster than light in a vacuum. As such, the speed of light in a vacuum will always be greater than the speed in any medium, so n must always be ≥1.000.

3. List the refractive index for different parts of the eye and for common lens materials.

See Table 1.1. It is likely not useful to memorize these, as you will almost always be given the refractive index if needed for a calculation (the only exception is that n = 1.000 for air). However, it is good to have a general idea of what these numbers are for different materials.

TABLE 1.1 ■ **Refractive Index of Various Materials**

Material	Refractive Index (n)
Air	1.000
Water	1.333
Aqueous/vitreous humor	1.336
Cornea	1.376
Acrylic	1.460
Polymethylmethacrylate (PMMA)	1.492
Crown glass	1.523

4. What happens when light crosses an interface at a perpendicular angle?

The light changes speed but does not change direction.

The change in speed depends on the difference in refractive indexes between the two materials. The higher the refractive index, the slower light travels through that material. As such, if light goes from a lower to a higher refractive index material, it slows down. Conversely, if light goes from a higher to a lower refractive index material, it speeds up (Fig. 1.2).

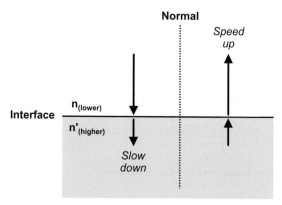

Direction does *not* change when light rays are parallel to the normal

Fig. 1.2   If light crosses an interface parallel to the normal (i.e., perpendicular to the interface), it changes speed but not direction.

If light strikes perpendicular to the interface, it does not change direction. By convention in geometric optics, all angles are measured relative to the *normal vector* (defined as a line perpendicular to the interface).

5. What happens when light crosses an interface at an angle?

The light changes speed and refracts (i.e., bends).

The direction in which the light bends depends on the difference in refractive indexes between the media. When light goes from:

Lower to higher refractive index → light bends *toward* the normal
Higher to lower refractive index → light bends *away* from the normal

One way to try to understand this is to think of a line of soldiers marching on smooth pavement next to tall grass. As the soldiers at one end begin marching in the grass, they are slowed down, and the line of soldiers is bent toward the normal (Fig. 1.3). Conversely, light is bent away from the normal when passing from a material with a higher index of refraction to a material with a lower one.

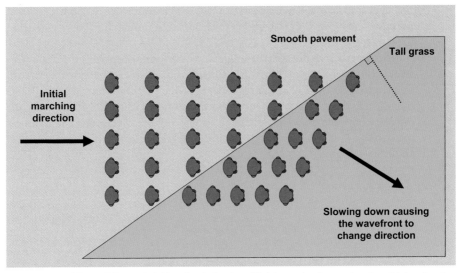

Fig. 1.3 Marching soldiers mimicking the behavior of light passing from a low to a high refractive index material.

6. What law determines how light is refracted at an interface?

Snell's law—The mathematical formula (n sin Ø = n' sin Ø') that describes how light is refracted at an interface (Fig. 1.4).

$$n \sin ø = n' \sin ø'$$

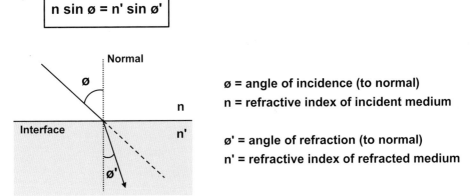

ø = angle of incidence (to normal)
n = refractive index of incident medium

ø' = angle of refraction (to normal)
n' = refractive index of refracted medium

Fig. 1.4 Snell's law.

7. What is the critical angle? Calculate the critical angle for the interface between crown glass (n = 1.52) and air.

The *critical angle* is the angle at which light is bent 90 degrees away from the normal. The critical angle is 41 degrees for the interface between crown glasses and air.

When light travels from a material with a higher refractive index to one with a lower refractive index, the light ray is bent away from the normal (i.e., more parallel to the refractive surface).

The critical angle is defined as the angle at which light is bent exactly 90 degrees away from the normal (Fig. 1.5). The critical angle can be calculated with Snell's law by using the refractive indexes of the two materials (n and n′), setting ø′ = 90 degrees, and solving for ø. For example, the critical angle for the interface between crown glass and air is determined by plugging the numbers into Snell's law: 1.52 sin ø = 1.00 sin 90 degrees. Solving for ø, the critical angle is 41 degrees.

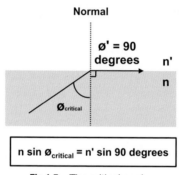

$$n \sin ø_{critical} = n' \sin 90 \text{ degrees}$$

Fig.1.5   The critical angle.

8. What is total internal reflection?

When the angle of incidence exceeds the critical angle (ø > ø$_{critical}$), the light is not refracted, but rather it is reflected back into the material with the higher refractive index. This is called *total internal reflection* (Fig. 1.6). Note that, as with all mirrors, the angle of reflection ø′ equals the angle of incidence ø (see Question 11).

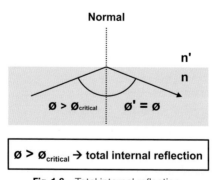

$$ø > ø_{critical} \rightarrow \text{total internal reflection}$$

Fig. 1.6   Total internal reflection.

EXAM PEARL

The critical angle and total internal reflection have meaning only when light bends *away* from the normal, so it only applies when light goes from a *higher* to *lower* refractive index material. Clinically, this is the reason you cannot see the anterior chamber angle directly. As light passes from the angle through the aqueous, cornea, tears, and air, it undergoes total internal reflection at the *tear–air* interface (*not* the *cornea–tear* interface). This is overcome with gonioscopy lenses, which replace the tear–air interface with a tear–plastic interface (less the difference in refractive index), allowing light from the angle to escape. Once escaped, the light is reflected by a mirror so that it exits the plastic (plastic–air interface) at an angle that is less than the critical angle (Fig. 1.7).

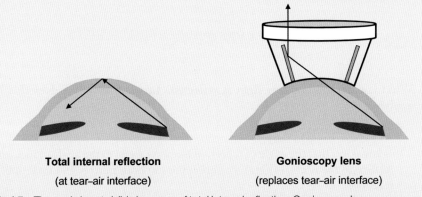

Total internal reflection

(at tear–air interface)

Gonioscopy lens

(replaces tear–air interface)

Fig. 1.7 The angle is not visible because of total internal reflection. Gonioscopy lenses overcome this by replacing the tear–air interface with a tear–plastic interface, allowing light to escape.

9. What is the difference between refraction and reflection?

Refraction is the bending of light at an interface as it passes from one transparent medium into another. *Reflection* is the bouncing of light off of a surface. In refraction, light traverses two different media, while in reflection, light stays within the same medium.

10. Can refraction and reflection both occur at the same interface?

Yes!

At any interface between two transparent surfaces, light rays can be both reflected and refracted. A good example in ophthalmology is the anterior surface of the cornea, which refracts light as a positive lens (refracting power ≅ +48 diopters) and reflects light as a negative mirror (reflecting power ≅ −255 diopters).

EXAM PEARL

The anterior surface of the cornea has a convex shape and can act as both a plus power lens and minus power mirror. For any optics question about corneal power, be careful to check whether the question is asking about the *refracting* power (high plus lens) or the *reflecting* power (high minus mirror) of the cornea (Fig. 1.8).

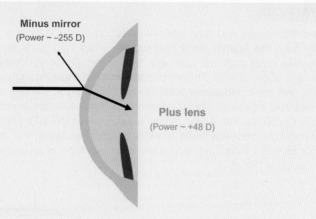

Fig. 1.8 Power of the anterior surface of the cornea, plus lens and minus mirror.

11. What law determines how light is reflected? In what scenarios does this law apply?

The law of reflection.

This law states that the angle of reflection is always equal to the angle of incidence, relative to the normal (Fig. 1.9). This applies to both mirrors and total internal reflection.

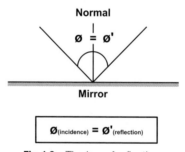

Fig. 1.9 The law of reflection.

CHAPTER 2

Vergence, Lenses, Objects, and Images

1. What is the definition of vergence? What is a diopter?

Vergence is the amount of spreading apart (or coming together) of a bundle of light rays. Vergence is positive if the light rays are converging (coming together), negative if the rays are diverging (spreading apart), and zero if the rays are parallel (Fig. 2.1). You can think of *divergence* (*negative vergence*) as light rays spreading apart from a single point, and *convergence* (*positive vergence*) as light rays coming together toward a single point.

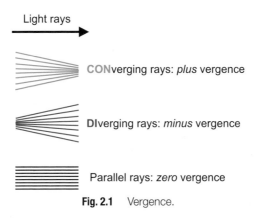

Light rays

CONverging rays: *plus* vergence

DIverging rays: *minus* vergence

Parallel rays: *zero* vergence

Fig. 2.1 Vergence.

A *diopter* (D) is the reciprocal of the distance (in meters), measured from the point where light rays intersect (i.e., the point where diverging light rays are coming from or the point where converging rays are going toward).

2. What is the formula for the power of a lens? What is the power of a diverging lens with a focal length of 5 cm?

The power of a lens:

$$P\,(\text{diopters}) = \frac{1}{\text{focal length}\,(\text{m})}$$

For a lens with a 5-cm focal length, the power is $P = 1/0.05$ m $= 20$ D (remember to convert cm to m). By convention, a diverging lens is negative, so $P = -20$ D.

EXAM PEARL

Many questions require that you convert a distance to a vergence (or vice versa). Remember, vergence is always the reciprocal of distance (vergence = 1/distance), and vice versa. Distances are often given in centimeters or millimeters, so be careful to convert to meters before taking the reciprocal. Also keep in mind that vergence is measured in diopters (D). Despite the similarity in name, *diopters* (D) are completely different from *prism diopters*, which are used in prisms (see Chapter 16, Prisms and Diplopia).

3. **What is the focal length of a +5 D lens? Where is its primary focal point? What about the secondary focal point? Where are the primary and secondary focal points for a −5 D lens?**

   Power: $P = 1/f \rightarrow f = 1/P = 1/5 \text{ D} = 0.20 \text{ m} = 20 \text{ cm focal length}$

   The *primary focal point* is the point along the optical axis at which an object must be placed for parallel rays to emerge from the lens. The primary focal point is to the left of a converging (plus) lens and to the right of a diverging (minus) lens (Figs. 2.2 and 2.3).

   Plus lens (+5 D)

   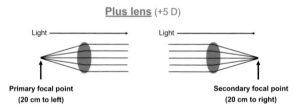

   Fig. 2.2   Primary and secondary focal points of a plus lens.

   Minus lens (−5 D)

   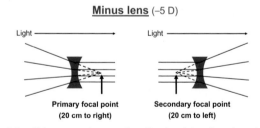

   Fig. 2.3   Primary and secondary focal points of a minus lens.

   The *secondary focal point* is the point along the optical axis where incoming parallel rays are brought into focus. The secondary focal point is to the right of a converging (plus) lens and to the left of a diverging (minus) lens (Figs. 2.2 and 2.3).

4. **What is the basic lens formula? What do each of the components represent?**

   The basic lens formula defines the relationships between an object, lens, and image. It is one of the most important equations in geometric optics (and optics exams) (Fig. 2.4).

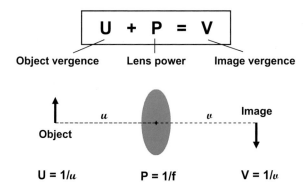

Upper case **U** and **V** represent vergences (in diopters)

Lower case u and v represent distances (in m)

Fig. 2.4 The basic lens formula.

5. **An object is located 2 m to the left of a +3 D lens (Fig. 2.5).**

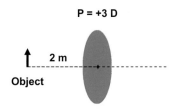

Fig. 2.5 Diagram of the lens system.

(a) **Where will the image be located for the lens system in Fig. 2.5?**

The image will be 40 cm to the right of the lens.

U = −1/2 m = −0.5 D (negative because light diverges from a real object)

$$U + P = V$$
$$(-0.5) + (+3) = V$$
$$V = -0.5 + 3 = +2.5 \text{ D}$$

V is positive, which means the image rays are converging as they emerge from the lens. This means that the light rays will intersect to the right of the lens, which is where the image is located.

$v = 1/2.5$ D = +0.40 m → The image is 40 cm to the right of the lens.

Light always diverges from real objects (which applies to most optics questions). *For real objects, object vergence is always negative (U < 0).* A positive object vergence can only be created by an optical system with multiple lenses/mirrors (or if you are specifically told that the object vergence is positive by a mean examiner).

> **(b) Is the image in question 5(a) real or virtual? How do you distinguish between real and virtual images when evaluating a lens system?**
>
> *It is a real image.*
>
> A real image is always on the same side of the lens as the actual rays of light forming the image (i.e., the image rays intersect to form the image). A virtual image must be located by imaginary extensions of the light rays into the object space. The same is true of real and virtual objects.

By convention, in geometric optics, light always goes from left to right. The object rays are always on the left of the lens, and the image rays are always on the right of the lens. An image (or object) is real if it is on the same side as the rays that define it, and virtual if it is on the opposite side. So, for any single-lens questions, you can generally assume:

Object: Real if on the left of the lens, virtual if on the right of the lens.

Image: Real if on the right of the lens, virtual if on the left of the lens.

Note, this is different for mirrors (see Chapter 3, Mirrors, for comparison chart).

> **(c) For the image in question 5(a), what is the transverse magnification? If the object is 10 cm tall, how tall is the image? Is the image upright or inverted relative to the object?**
>
> *The transverse magnification = −1/5. The image is 2 cm tall and inverted.*
>
> Transverse magnification is equal to $\frac{\text{image size}}{\text{object size}}$ which is proportional to $\frac{\text{image distance}}{\text{object distance}}$. Since distance = 1/vergence, this is equal to $\frac{\text{image distance}=1/V}{\text{object distance}=1/U} = \frac{U}{V}$. Note that since you have a reciprocal over a reciprocal, you end up with the slightly counterintuitive result that even though magnification is image distance over object distance, the transverse magnification formula is equal to object vergence over image vergence. If that is too complicated, just memorize the following:
>
> The formula for transverse magnification is:
>
> $$\boxed{\text{Mag} = U/V \text{ (object vergence/image vergence)}}$$
>
> For this question, transverse magnification is calculated as:
>
> $$\text{Mag} = -0.5/2.5 = -1/5$$

$$\text{Image size} = \text{Object size} \times \text{Mag}$$
$$= 10 \text{ cm} \times -1/5$$
$$= -2 \text{ cm} \rightarrow \text{the image is 2 cm high}$$

Since the magnification is negative, the image is inverted.

EXAM PEARL

There are two ways to determine the orientation of an image (i.e., upright vs inverted).
1. Draw a ray diagram; only the central ray is needed.
2. Use the sign of the magnification: Mag > 0 → image upright, Mag < 0 → image inverted. Be careful with the signs of U and V (remember that U is always negative for real objects), as this information is needed to calculate the orientation correctly.

---

6. **Calculate the vergence at 10 cm, 40 cm, and 10 m from a real object.**

The vergences are −10 D (at 10 cm), –2.5 D (at 40 cm), and –0.1 D (at 10 m) (Fig. 2.6).

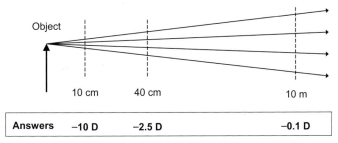

Fig. 2.6   Answer to Question 6.

The vergence is the inverse of the distance (in meters) from the object. Remember to convert the distances to meters. So, $\frac{1}{0.1} = 10$ D, $\frac{1}{0.4} = 2.5$ D, and $\frac{1}{10} = 0.1$ D. Since real objects always produce negative vergence (the rays are diverging), the vergences are all negative.

7. **Parallel rays of light pass through a +1 D lens. Calculate the vergence of light at 25 cm, 90 cm, and 125 cm from the lens.**

The vergences are +1.33 D (at 25 cm), +10 D (at 90 cm), and –4 D (at 125 cm) (Fig. 2.7).

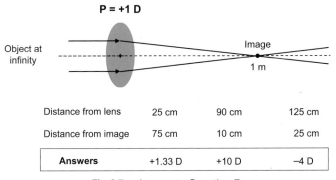

Fig. 2.7   Answer to Question 7.

Remember, parallel rays of light have a vergence of zero (object vergence: $U = 0$). To calculate the position of the image, use $U + P = V$:

$$U + P = V$$
$$0 + 1 = V$$
$$V = 1$$

$v = 1/V = 1/1 = 1$ m → the image distance is 1 m.

The image is formed where light rays intersect, which is 1 m to the right of the lens (vergence is infinity at the point of intersection). The vergence along the path of light is calculated by taking the inverse of the distance to the *image*. (A beginner might mistakenly calculate the distance from the *lens*.) To the left of the image, the rays are converging so the vergences are positive. To the right of the image, the rays are diverging so the vergences are negative.

8. **Light from a distant star passes through a −1 D lens. Where is the image? What is the vergence of the image rays 1 m to the left of the lens, 25 cm to the left of the lens, and 25 cm to the right of the lens?**

   The image is 1 m to the left of the lens. The vergences are infinity (at 1 m to the left), −1.33 D (at 25 cm to the left), and −0.8 D (at 25 cm to the right) (Fig. 2.8).

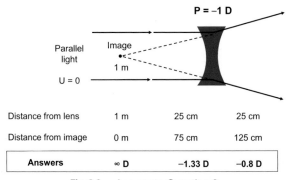

Fig. 2.8   Answer to Question 8.

Light from a distant star is far enough away that it can be considered to originate from infinity so that the rays are parallel; that is, $U = 0$.

$$U + P = V$$
$$(0) + (-1) = V$$
$$V = -1 \, D$$
$$v = 1/V = 1/-1 = -1 \, m$$

Since the rays have minus vergence when leaving the lens, the image rays diverge and will never meet to the right of the lens. Imaginary lines must be drawn back toward the source of light to find the point of intersection. Thus the image must be located at some distance to the left of the lens. To determine how far to the left, take a reciprocal:

The image is located $\frac{1}{-1\,D}$ = −1 m, or 1 m to the left of the lens.

1 m to the left of the lens is the exact location of the image. Where the lines intersect, vergence is infinite (∞).

25 cm to the left of the lens is 75 cm to the right of the image. At this point, the rays are diverging, so vergence = −1/0.75 m = −1.33 D.

25 cm to the right of the lens is 125 cm to the right of the image. At this point, the rays are diverging, so vergence = −1/1.25 m = −0.8 D.

EXAM PEARL

When calculating vergence, remember a few important points:
1. Except for parallel rays of light, the vergence of light rays does not remain constant. It changes continuously and is calculated by taking the reciprocal of the distance to the point of intersection.
2. The farther away the point of intersection, the closer the vergence will be to 0 (i.e., the light rays get more parallel as they approach infinity). If a question says that an object is very far away or that light is coming from a distant star, you can assume the light is very close to parallel, and vergence = 0 for calculations.

9. **Where is the image for an object located to the left of an +8 D lens at a distance of:**

(a) **100 cm**

(b) **50 cm**

(c) **250 mm**

(d) **12.5 cm**

(e) **0.011 m**

What is the transverse magnification for each image and is it upright or inverted?

See Table 2.1.

TABLE 2.1 ■ **Answer to Question 9**

	Image Location	Transverse Mag	Upright/Inverted
(a)	14.3 cm	−0.14	Inverted
	U = −1/100 cm = −1/1 m = −1 D (diverging)	M = U/V	M < 0 → inverted
	U + P = V	M = −1/7	
	−1 + 8 = V	M = −0.14	
	V = +7		
	v = 1/V = 1/7		
	v = +0.143 m = 14.3 cm to the right of the lens		

(Continued)

TABLE 2.1 ■ Answer to Question 9 *(cont'd)*

	Image Location	Transverse Mag	Upright/Inverted
(b)	16.7 cm	−0.33	Inverted
(c)	25 cm	−1.00	Inverted
(d)	Infinity	Undefined	-
	(V = 0 → zero vergence, parallel rays of light)		
(e)	−1.2 cm	+1.1	Upright
			M > 0 → upright

10. **Recalculate the answers in question 9 if the lens had a power of −8 D (instead of +8 D).**

   See Table 2.2.

TABLE 2.2 ■ Answer to Question 10

10.	Image Location	Transverse Mag	Upright/Inverted
(a)	−11.1 cm	0.11	Upright
(b)	−10 cm	0.20	Upright
(c)	−8.3 cm	0.33	Upright
(d)	−6.25 cm	0.50	Upright
(e)	−1.0 cm	0.92	Upright

EXAM PEARL

The first rule of optics is: *When in doubt, take a reciprocal.* Many questions in optics require you to take reciprocals, often several. To help minimize mistakes:

1. Make sure you look at the units carefully. For instance, a measurement in millimeters or centimeters needs to be converted to meters before you calculate the reciprocal to get a vergence or power in diopters.
2. Many high-stakes exams do not allow calculators. You will still be asked to calculate simple reciprocals, so it is useful to know how to calculate these quickly in your head or memorize common reciprocals (Table 2.3). Just tape this handy table to your bathroom mirror a week before the exam and you will be suffused with a sense of invincibility as you start to take the test. Or not, but it will be one less thing to worry about.

TABLE 2.3 ■ Simple Reciprocals (Most Common in Bold)

1/1	**1**	**1/8**	**0.125**
1/2	**0.50**	1/9	0.11
1/3	**0.33**	**1/10**	**0.10**
1/4	**0.25**	1/11	0.09
1/5	**0.20**	**1/12**	**0.08**
1/6	0.17	**1/20**	**0.05**
1/7	0.14	**1/25**	**0.04**

11. **An object is located 10 cm to the left of a +1 D lens, which is 14 cm to the left of a +5 D lens.**

   (a) Where is the image relative to the object?

   (b) Is it real or virtual?

   (c) What is the transverse magnification?

   (d) Is the image upright or inverted?

Answers:
(a) The image is 1.24 m to the right of the object
(b) Real
(c) Mag = −4.4
(d) Inverted

It is helpful to first draw a diagram (Fig. 2.9) and then solve each lens system separately.

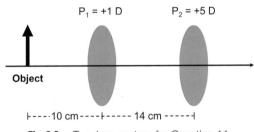

$P_1 = +1\,D$ $P_2 = +5\,D$

Object

|----10 cm----|----- 14 cm -----|

Fig. 2.9   Two-lens system for Question 11.

$u_1 = -10\ \text{cm} = -0.1\ \text{m}$ $u_2 = 11+14\ \text{cm} = 25\ \text{cm to the left of } P_2 = -0.25\ \text{m}$

$U_1 = 1/-0.1\ \text{m} = -10\ D$ $U_2 = 1/-0.25 = -4\ D$

$U_1 + P_1 = V_1$ $U_2 + P_2 = V_2$

$-10+1 = V_1$ $-4+5 = V_2$

$V_1 = -9\ D$ $V_2 = +1$

$v_1 = 1/-9 = -0.11\ \text{m}$ $v_2 = 1/1 = 1\ \text{m}$

   (a) Image is 1 m to the right of the +5 D lens, thus the image is 1 m + 10 cm + 14 cm = 124 cm = 1.24 m to the right of the object

   (b) Image is to the right of the final lens → on the same side of the lens as the rays that define it → real image

$$\text{Mag}_1 = U_1/V_1 = -10/-9 \qquad \text{Mag}_2 = U_2/V_2 = -4/1$$

$$\text{Mag}_1 = 1.11 \qquad\qquad\qquad \text{Mag}_2 = -4$$

(c) $\text{Mag}_{\text{total}} = \text{Mag}_1 \times \text{Mag}_2 = 1.11 \times -4 = -4.4\text{x}$

(d) $\text{Mag}_{\text{total}} < 0 \rightarrow$ Image is inverted

EXAM PEARL

For multiple-lens systems, answer the question by following the path of light, treating the lenses one at a time, sequentially, from left to right. The image of the first lens (Image 1) is the same as the object of the second lens (Object 2). The first lens is then ignored when performing the basic lens equation for the second lens (Image 2).

Location: The final image location (the final v) is relative to the last lens in the system. Be careful, the questioner may ask where the final image is relative to the object or a different lens in the system.

Magnification: To calculate the total magnification of the system, calculate the magnification of each lens system separately and then multiply them together: $\text{Mag}_{\text{total}} = \text{Mag}_1 \times \text{Mag}_2 \times \dots$

Orientation: Be careful with the signs during magnification calculations. The final magnification can tell you if the image is upright (Mag > 0) or inverted (Mag < 0) relative to the object. Alternatively, if you draw a central ray for each lens system, you can visualize whether each image is upright or inverted.

12. **For the following lens system (Fig. 2.10), please determine the following characteristics:**

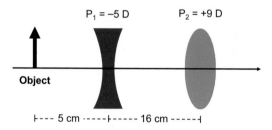

Fig. 2.10   Two-lens system for Question 12.

(a) **Where is the final image relative to the +9 D lens?**

(b) **Is it real or virtual?**

(c) **What is the transverse magnification?**

(d) **Is the final image upright or inverted?**

Answers:
(a) Image location is 25 cm to the right of the +9 D lens
(b) Real
(c) Transverse magnification = −1
(d) Inverted

13. **You are eating a peanut butter and jelly sandwich and drop a large, perfectly smooth, hemispherical glob of jelly. The jelly has an index of refraction of 1.33. The radius of the curvature of the glob is 25 mm. What is the refractive power of the surface where jelly meets air?**

The refractive power P = +13.2 D (Fig. 2.11).

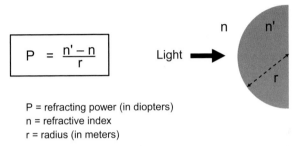

$$P = \frac{n' - n}{r}$$

P = refracting power (in diopters)
n = refractive index
r = radius (in meters)

Fig. 2.11   The formula for refracting power for a spherical refracting surface.

In this case, n′ = 1.33, n = 1.00 (for air), and r = 0.025 m.
Thus the power is: P = (1.33 − 1)/0.025 = +13.2 D (positive power because the medium with the higher refractive index has a convex surface).

EXAM PEARL

To determine if a single refracting surface has positive or negative power, draw a box around the surface and then color in the side of the box that has the higher refractive index. The colored-in area will now look like a lens, and the lens will look like a plus/plano or minus/plano lens (Fig. 2.12).

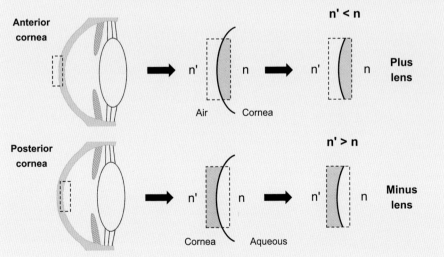

Fig. 2.12   Method to determine the power of a single refracting surface. (Note: Refractive index of cornea is 1.376; refractive index of aqueous is 1.336.)

14. **Before leaving for a scuba diving trip in Hawaii, you pack your favorite +20 D indirect ophthalmoscopy lens in your suitcase ($n_{glass} = 1.52$), because as a budding retina surgeon, you never go anywhere without it. While scuba diving, you decide to use your lens to get a closer look at the scales of a most interesting fish. What is the power of the +20 D lens underwater ($n_{water} = 1.33$)? (You may assume you are holding an ideal thin lens.)**

Lens power under water : $P = +7.3\ D$

The refracting power of a thin lens is proportional to the difference in refractive index between the lens and the medium. Since the radius of the curvature does not change when the lens is plunged underwater, it does not need to be included in the equation.

$$\frac{P_{air}}{P_{water}} = \frac{n_{lens} - n_{air}}{n_{lens} - n_{water}}$$

Filling in what is known:

$$\frac{20\ D}{P_{water}} = \frac{1.52 - 1.00}{1.52 - 1.33} = 2.73$$

$$P_{water} = \frac{20\ D}{2.73} = +7.3\ D$$

CHAPTER 3

Mirrors

1. **A frugal, dapper, 160-cm-tall ophthalmologist wishes to purchase a mirror that he will mount on the wall to view his entire outfit before heading to the office. He must choose from among 1-m, 2-m, and 3-m mirrors. Which is the shortest (thus the least expensive) mirror he can purchase to get the job done? Is his image real or virtual?**

   He should purchase the 1-m mirror. The image is virtual.

   The light ray heading from the bottom of his foot to his eye will reflect off the mirror at a point half the distance from his foot to his eye, or 80 cm above the level of the foot. No mirror is required below that point. If the top of the mirror is precisely at eye level, only an 80-cm mirror is needed, so the 1-m mirror will work (leaving a little extra room to allow him to mount the mirror above eye level so he can also check out his awesome hair.)

   A plano mirror reverses the direction of the light without changing vergence, and therefore it has zero power. The image formed of a real object by a plano mirror is always virtual, upright, the same size as the object, and the same distance behind the mirror as the object is in front of it (Fig. 3.1).

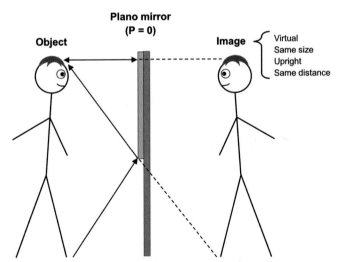

Fig. 3.1 Plano mirror; only needs to be half the height of the person to see the entire body.

2. A concave mirror has a radius of curvature of 25 cm. What is the power of the mirror?

> *The power of the mirror is +8 D.*

As with a lens, the reflecting power of a mirror is equal to the reciprocal of the focal length, P = 1/f. Since f = r/2, to calculate the power using the radius of curvature, we use the formula: P = −2/r (Fig. 3.2).

$$P_{reflecting} = \frac{1}{f} = -\frac{2}{r}$$

f = focal length (m)

r = radius of curvature (m)

Fig. 3.2 Reflecting power of a mirror.

The negative sign in front of the −2/r is needed to follow convention. For the problems we will be asked to solve, to determine whether the mirror has positive or negative power, it is easiest to just look at whether it is concave (plus power) or convex (minus power) (Fig. 3.3).

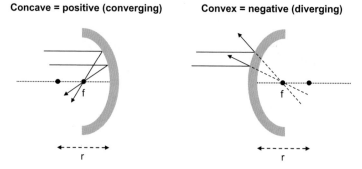

Concave = positive (converging)   **Convex = negative (diverging)**

Fig. 3.3 Concave versus convex mirrors.

Power = 2/r = 2/0.25 m = 8 → +8 D (plus power because the mirror is concave).

3. What part of the eye is used as a convex mirror in ophthalmic instrumentation? What other tests depend on this part of the eye acting as a convex mirror?

> The front surface of the cornea (technically the tear film) is used as a convex mirror in manual keratometry and corneal topography. Tests of ocular alignment (Krimsky and Hirschberg tests) also depend on the corneal light reflex produced by this convex mirror function.

4. The anterior surface of a cornea has a reflecting power of −250 D. What is the radius of curvature? What is the estimated refracting power of the anterior surface of the cornea (assuming n of the cornea = 1.376)? What about the estimated refracting power of the cornea as a whole (using an averaged corneal refractive index of 1.3375 to account for the front and back surfaces)?

The radius of curvature is 8 mm and the estimated refracting powers are +47 D (anterior cornea) and +42 D (cornea as a whole).

To calculate the radius of curvature, use the mirror power formula, $P = -2/r$. Then, $r = -2/P = 0.008$ m $= 8$ mm.

Remember, the front of the cornea acts as both a positive *refractive* surface (i.e., lens) for most of the light passing through it and as a negative (convex) *reflective* surface (i.e., mirror) for the small percentage of light that is reflected. The radius of curvature of the cornea can be used for both calculations. Now that you know the radius of curvature, you can calculate the refractive power of the anterior surface of the cornea using the equation for the refractive power of a single surface.

$$P_{anterior\ cornea} = (n' - n)/r = (1.376 - 1)/0.008 = 47 = +47\ D$$

This is essentially how a manual keratometer works—it uses the *reflective* power of the cornea to measure the radius of the cornea and then uses the radius to estimate the *refractive* power. The reason we use the keratometric index of refraction (1.3375) instead of the exact refractive index of the cornea (1.376) is to account for the negative refractive power of the posterior cornea.

$$P_{cornea} = (n' - n)/r = (1.3375 - 1)/0.008 = 42.2 = +42\ D$$

5. **A transilluminator light source ("muscle light") is held 10 cm in front of a cornea that has a reflecting power of −250 D.**

   (a) **Where is the image of the light source?**

   The image is 3.8 mm behind the cornea (Fig. 3.4).

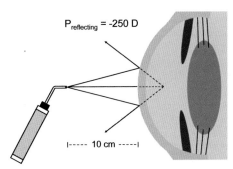

Fig. 3.4 Mirror diagram for the anterior surface of the cornea.

For mirror calculations, as with lens calculations, we can use the formula $U + P = V$, except that the light changes direction after striking the mirror.
$U = 1/object\ distance = 1/0.10$ m $= -10$ D (minus because light *always* diverges from a real object)
$P = -250$ D (given in question)

$$U + P = V$$
$$(-10) + (-250) = V$$

$V = -260\ D \rightarrow$ The negative value means that the reflected light is diverging as it reflects off the corneal surface. This means that the image is found by creating imaginary extensions of the rays of light behind the cornea (to the right of the cornea in the diagram). The distance of the image from the mirror (reflective surface on the front of the cornea) is the reciprocal of the vergence at the point of departure = $1/-260\ D = -0.0038\ m = 3.8\ mm$ behind the cornea.

(b) What is the magnification of the image of the light source?

Magnification = U/V = −10/−260 = +0.038

Note that you can also calculate magnification by dividing image distance/ object distance = *v/u* = 0.0038 m/0.10 m = +0.038.

(c) Is the image upright or inverted?

Upright.

If you keep track of signs when calculating magnification, the end result is a positive number (Mag = +0.038), so the image is upright. You can also ignore the signs by drawing a central ray from the tip of the object through the center of curvature of the mirror to visualize the end result using ray tracing (Fig. 3.5).

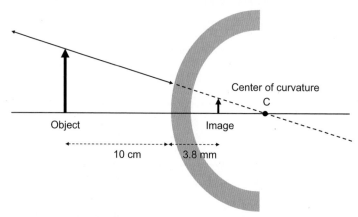

Fig. 3.5   Ray tracing. By drawing the central ray (from the tip of the object to the center of curvature of the mirror), you can determine that the image is upright (and minified).

(d) Is the image real or virtual?

Virtual.

The image is behind the mirror, on the opposite side of the mirror from the rays that define it, making it a virtual image.

6. For a convex mirror, what are the image characteristics of a real object?

For a convex (minus) mirror, such as the front of the cornea, the image of a real object is always virtual, erect (upright), and minified. (You can think of the mnemonic, "VErMin"—or not, if the idea of vermin crawling all over a convex mirror is not something you want to be dealing with.)

EXAM PEARL

For optics questions on *lenses* versus *mirrors*, there are important similarities and differences (Table 3.1).

TABLE 3.1 ■ Comparison of Characteristics Between Lenses and Mirrors

	Lenses	Mirrors
Formula	U (object vergence) + P (power) = V (image vergence)	
Magnification	Mag = image distance/object distance = U/V	
Image orientation	Mag > 0 → upright/Mag < 0 → inverted, or draw a central ray	
Central ray	Through the center of the lens	Through the center of curvature of the mirror
Object/image	Object (or image) is real when it is on the same side as the rays that define it	
Object rays	To the left of the lens and mirror	
Image rays	To the right of the lens	To the left of the mirror
Power magnitude	$P = 1/f = (n' - n)/r$	$P = 1/f = -2/r$ (plug $n' = -1$, $n = 1$ into lens power formula)
Power plus/minus	Concave negative/convex positive	Concave positive/convex negative

7. Louise Gross, an elite athlete, is checking her eye and notices a speck between two lashes. She is 10 cm from a plano mirror. How far away is the image of the speck from the mirror? How far is the image from Louise's eye?

The image is 10 cm from the mirror, 20 cm from Louise's eye.

For plano mirrors, the image is the same distance behind the mirror as the object is in front of it; therefore the image is 10 cm behind the mirror and 20 cm from Louise's eye.

This can also be calculated using the formula U + P = V (plano mirrors have zero power):

$$U + P = V$$
$$1/-0.1 + 0 = V$$
$$V = -10\,D$$

$$v = 1/-10\,D = -0.10\,m = 10\,cm \text{ behind the mirror}$$

Vergence leaving the mirror, V = -10 D, so the reflected light is diverging and the image will be somewhere to the right of (behind) the mirror. Distance from the mirror is 1/-10 D = 10 cm behind (to the right of) the mirror or 20 cm from Louise's eye.

8. **Concerned about the speck, Lousie flips her mirror over and looks into a concave mirror on the other side of the plano mirror. The concave mirror has a radius of curvature of 50 cm.**

    (a) **How far away from her eye is the image of the speck, which she now realizes is a louse?**

       The image is 26.7 cm from the eye (Fig. 3.6).

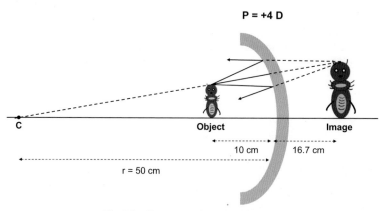

Fig. 3.6 Concave mirror ray diagram.

    The power of the concave mirror is $P = 2/r = 2/0.5$ m $= 4$ D ($+4$ D as the mirror is concave) (Fig. 3.6).

$$\text{Using } U + P = V$$

$$-10 + 4 = V$$

$$V = -6 \text{ D} \rightarrow \text{reflected light is diverging}$$

$$v = 1/-6 \text{ D} = -0.167 \text{ m} = 16.7 \text{ cm behind the mirror}$$

    The distance from the mirror $= 1/-6$ D $= -0.167$ m or 16.7 cm behind (to the right of) the mirror. Therefore the image is 16.7 cm behind the mirror, which is 10 cm from the eye, so the image is 26.7 cm from the eye.

    (b) **Is the image real or virtual?**

       Virtual.

       The image is behind the mirror, on the opposite side of the mirror from the rays that define it, so it is a virtual image.

    (c) **What is the transverse magnification of the louse?**

       Transverse magnification $= +1.67$.

Corresponding points of the object and image must fall on the central ray, so the image must be magnified (Fig. 3.6).

To calculate the transverse magnification: Mag = U/V = −10 D/− 6 D = +1.67

Or, Mag = image distance/object distance = −0.167 m/−0.10 m = +1.67

The number is greater than 1, so it is magnified.

(d) Is it inverted or upright?

Upright.

Corresponding points of the object and image must fall on the central ray, so the image must be upright (Fig. 3.6).

Also, the +1.67 magnification is > 0, which means that the image is upright.

CHAPTER 4

Principles of Light and Lasers

1. What is the difference between geometric optics and physical optics?

Geometric optics explains optical phenomena using light rays. The light rays travel along straight lines and do not change direction unless refracted (by a lens) or reflected (by a mirror). This is an artificial but mathematically useful construct that we use to perform lens and mirror calculations.

Physical optics deals with the wave and photon (particle) properties of light. Physical optics is needed to explain light phenomena in the physical world, such as scattering, polarization, interference, coherence, and diffraction.

2. What is light?

Visible light represents the narrow section of the electromagnetic spectrum that the human retina can detect. Light can be described in terms of speed (c), frequency (f), and wavelength (λ) using the equation, $c = f\lambda$. The speed of light in a vacuum is 3.0×10^8 m/s. The electromagnetic spectrum has a huge range of wavelengths, but human eyes can detect only a small portion of this energy, the visible spectrum, from 400 nm (near-ultraviolet) to 700 nm (near-infrared) (Fig. 4.1).

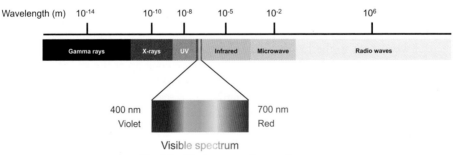

Fig. 4.1 Electromagnetic spectrum.

3. What is scattering? What are the three types of scattering?

Light can be described as either electromagnetic waves or particles. When considered particles, the particles of light interact with particles in the atmosphere as they travel toward their destination, with a resulting change in direction. This phenomenon is known as *scattering*. The type of scattering observed depends on the size of the particles the light interacts with.

1. *Rayleigh scattering* occurs when light interacts with particles much *smaller* than the wavelength of the light ("Rayleigh" → "really little"), such as gas

molecules in the atmosphere. The intensity of scattering is inversely proportional to the wavelength (to the fourth power), so it affects shorter wavelengths more. This explains why the sky is blue (see detailed explanation in Question 4) and the bluish appearance of the cornea and lens.

2. *Mie scattering* occurs when light interacts with particles the *same* size as the wavelength ("I am the same size as Mie") such as water droplets in clouds. The intensity does not vary greatly with wavelength, so all wavelengths are scattered equally. This explains why clouds are white and why cataracts appear white.

3. *Geometric scattering* occurs when light interacts with particles much *larger* than the wavelength ("Big GMC Sierra"). At this level, the interaction essentially follows the laws of geometric optics (i.e., refraction and reflection).

4. Why is the sky blue and why is the sun red/orange at sunset and sunrise?

Scattering. (Rayleigh scattering if you are looking for extra credit!)

At some point, most ophthalmologists will be asked this question (if not on an exam, then by colleagues or kids). The color of the sky is explained by the presence of particles—gas molecules—in the atmosphere. Consider first the images of men walking on the moon. Even with the sun visible, the sky is completely black because there are no gas molecules surrounding the moon to scatter the light into the observer's eye. Back on earth, light encounters gas molecules as it travels through the atmosphere, and *scattering* deflects the passing light toward the observer, making the light "visible." (Similarly, a projector beam is not normally visible in a theater but will become visible if there is dust or smoke in the room to scatter the light, though in that case the particles are larger and all wavelengths are scattered equally via *Mie* scattering.) The intensity of the light scattered by gas molecules in the atmosphere is inversely proportional to the wavelength to the fourth power, thus shorter (blue), high-energy wavelengths are scattered more. For this reason, when you look up at the sky at noon on a clear day, mostly blue light is scattered toward your eyes and the sky appears blue rather than black. Longer-wavelength light is scattered much less. The sun itself appears slightly yellow when viewed directly at noon, having lost mainly its blue components. At sunrise and sunset, the light reaching you has passed through more of the atmosphere and has "lost" its shorter-wavelength components; you see what is left over: the longer wavelengths (red and orange).

5. What fundamental characteristic of light is used to perform Titmus stereo testing?

Polarization.

When light energy is described as electromagnetic waves, the waves are composed of magnetic and electric fields oscillating perpendicular to each other. Polarization refers to the orientation of the electric field as the light travels toward its destination. Most visible light has randomly oriented electric fields; that is, it is unpolarized. If the orientation of the electric fields is not random, then the light is polarized. For example, if all electric fields of the light waves within a beam of light are oriented vertically, the light is said to be vertically polarized. There are other forms of polarization that you might hear about, such as circular or elliptical, but this is beyond the scope of clinical optics.

To create a three-dimensional effect with the Titmus stereo test (or other tests of binocular vision), slightly different objects must be projected to the two eyes. In the old days, this was accomplished using red and green objects, projected through red and green glasses. However, these stereoscopic images are devoid of color information. Modern tests, such as the Titmus stereo test, project objects that are linearly polarized 90 degrees away from each other; specifically, one object is polarized at 45 degrees, the other at 135 degrees. The observer wears glasses with polarized lenses (at similar orientations to the objects) over each eye. Each lens allows only the polarized rays from one image to pass; thus a different image passes through to each eye, and binocular vision and stereopsis are simulated.

6. Vertically polarized light is used to project a letter onto a screen. What happens to the image if a vertically oriented polarizing filter is placed in the path of light? What about when the polarizing filter is held horizontally?

Vertically polarized light will pass through a vertical polarizing filter virtually unchanged. In contrast, it will be completely blocked by a horizontal polarizing filter.

7. Why do polarizing glasses reduce reflections and glare?

When light is scattered (e.g., the blue sky) or reflected (e.g., off of the car ahead of you), it becomes partially polarized. The axis of polarization of the scattered and reflected light is usually horizontal. Polarized sunglasses use vertical polarizing filters that block this predominantly horizontal component of reflected and scattered light.

8. What optical phenomena are the basis of antireflection coatings?

Coherence and interference.

Interference occurs when two distinct light waves emerge from a single source and then overlap. If the peaks of the light waves overlap, they will add to each other to create areas of maximum intensity (constructive interference). If the peak of one wave matches the valley of the other, the light is extinguished (destructive interference). This alternation of light and dark areas is known as an interference pattern.

Coherence is simply a measure of the ability of two light beams to interfere with each other. If all the waves in a beam of light have peaks that align, that beam of light has high coherence.

Antireflection coatings are 1/4 wavelength thick. Light rays are reflected at both the air/coating interface and the coating/glass interface, emerging exactly 1/2 wavelength out of phase. As such, the peak of one reflected wave matches the valley of another, producing destructive interference (Fig. 4.2). That is, if the reflected light wave from the front surface of the coating hits a "valley" just as the reflected light wave from the back surface of the coating hits a "peak," the net reflection will be nothing. Different coatings are required for different wavelengths of light. When spectacle lenses have antireflection coatings, the complex coatings required to reduce reflections of all wavelengths cause the reflections that do emerge to have a multicolored "rainbow" hue.

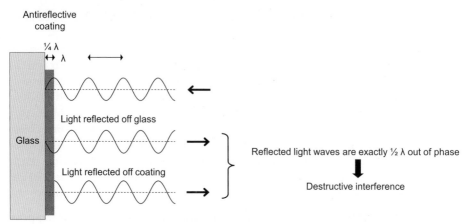

Fig. 4.2 Antireflection coating; ¼ λ thickness creates destructive interference in reflected light.

9. **What light phenomenon explains why image quality can be affected by a small pupil? At what pupil size does this begin to limit visual acuity?**

Diffraction.

Diffraction begins to affect vision when the pupil is less than 2.5 mm in diameter. Any light ray is bent slightly when it encounters an obstruction or aperture. This is known as *diffraction*. The smaller the size of the aperture, the greater the spreading of light caused by diffraction. An aperture of less than 2.5 mm (e.g., the pupil of the eye) begins to cause enough spreading to affect visual acuity. This is different from the optimal size of a pinhole to correct refractive error (i.e., 1.2 mm; see Chapter 6, Visual Acuity Testing).

EXAM PEARL

Some characteristics of light change with different wavelengths of light. It is important to keep clear in your mind which phenomena change, how they change, and their clinical relevance.
1. *Refraction* increases with *shorter* (high energy) wavelengths ("Blue Bends Better"). This causes chromatic aberration. Think of the high-energy blue light as more reactive, while the relaxed, low-energy red light just glides through the lens without bending as much.
2. *Scattering* (Rayleigh scattering) increases with *shorter* wavelengths. This is why the sky is blue during the day, as shorter blue light rays scatter and become visible, and red at sunset, as most of the shorter wavelengths have been scattered away. Again, the relaxed red light is not interested in getting scattered whereas the intense blue light is bouncing all over the place. You probably have friends like that.
3. *Diffraction* increases with *longer* wavelengths. The relaxed red light is distracted by the aperture edge and bends around to see what is going on, while the intense blue light is focused on getting through the aperture to get to its appointment on time.
4. *Reflection* does *not change* with different wavelengths of light.

10. What are radiometry and photometry?

Radiometry is the measurement of the amount of light produced by a source or illuminating a surface (measured in watts).

Photometry measures the power of light in terms of the responsiveness of the eye (measured in candelas, lumens, or lux, depending on how the light is being characterized).

11. During your comprehensive ophthalmology clinic, you examine Hal Lloyd, a 55-year-old diabetic man, and discover that he has severe asteroid hyalosis, making it almost impossible to see his retina. Mr. Lloyd has 20/20 corrected visual acuity. Why doesn't he complain of decreased vision? You are concerned that he might have early diabetic retinopathy. How will you examine his retina?

In asteroid hyalosis, "asteroids" (accumulations of calcium soaps in the vitreous) are small, dense opacities that cast tiny shadows (umbral cones) and reduce the total amount of light reaching the retina. The opacities also scatter a small portion of the light, but they do not reduce acuity because the umbral cones are so short that they do not reach the retina. Patients are thus rarely aware of asteroid hyalosis, and it is extremely uncommon that visual acuity is diminished. The ophthalmoscopic appearance of asteroid hyalosis is striking because so much light is reflected back toward the observer by the asteroids. The scattering causes glare that makes it difficult to visualize the retina.

There are now several options to examine the retina in asteroid hyalosis. Fluorescein angiography can be used. Since the yellow-green fluorescent light "source" is inside the eye, reflections and glare are not a problem for the observer. Ultrasonography, which does not depend on light rays, can also be used. Unfortunately, both of these techniques have relatively lower resolution compared to indirect ophthalmoscopy. In contrast, scanning laser ophthalmoscopy and optical coherence tomography provide retinal images with excellent resolution in asteroid hyalosis. Both approaches use methods that filter out almost all scattered light by precise selection of the targeted focal plane.

12. What does "laser" stand for? What are the three basic components of a laser?

Laser stands for "light amplification by stimulated emission of radiation." The three basic ingredients of a laser are:
1. A power source to supply energy (the *pump*)
2. An active medium with special properties that can generate light energy by emitting photons (the *contents*)
3. A chamber with mirrors at opposite ends to reflect the energy back and forth, one of which is partially transmitting (the *chamber*)

13. What is so special about laser light?

Laser light is characterized by certain properties; think of the properties of light in this chapter:
1. Monochromatic (single wavelength)
2. Polarized (all electric waves are oriented in the same direction)
3. Coherent (in phase; capable of creating interference when two beams interact)

  4. Unidirectional (nonspreading)
  5. High intensity (capable of delivering a lot of energy to a very small area)

14. **How does laser light interact with tissue? Name five distinct mechanisms and give an example of each.**

  See Table 4.1.

TABLE 4.1 ■ Types of Lasers With Interaction Type, Mechanism, and Examples

Interaction Type	Mechanism	Examples
Photochemical interaction (photoactivation)	Laser interacts with a photosensitizing dye to cause a photochemical reaction	Photodynamic therapy (PDT)
Photocoagulation (thermal interaction)	Laser absorption increases temperature and causes thermal damage (tissue must absorb the particular wavelength)	Argon, krypton
Photoablation	Laser breaks covalent bonds with UV light	Excimer
Plasma-induced ablation	Laser strips electrons leading to plasma formation	Femtosecond
Photodisruption	Laser generates a shock wave	Nd:YAG

15. **Are argon/krypton lasers operated continuously or pulsed? What about the neodymium:yttrium-aluminum-garnet (Nd:YAG) laser? Why is the power set in watts for some lasers and joules for others?**

  Argon and krypton photocoagulation lasers operate continuously while the Nd:YAG laser is pulsed. A joule is a watt of energy delivered for 1 second. Since continuous lasers vary in time of delivery, the total energy (in joules) cannot be known beforehand, and the power is set in watts (joules per second). Pulsed lasers deliver energy in a very short burst, so the total energy of each burst can be measured and the power is set in joules.

16. **A patient has a retinal tear that is just visible through a vitreous hemorrhage. What type of laser (color/wavelength) would be best to use?**

  A red laser (e.g., krypton red, wavelength 647 mm) is poorly absorbed by hemoglobin but well absorbed by melanin (retinal pigment epithelium (RPE), choroid), so it is ideal for lasering the retina through vitreous hemorrhage.

17. **What is special about the mechanism of action of a diode laser?**

  A diode laser operates in the infrared range and is not absorbed by any ocular contents other than melanin. During treatment, melanin absorbs the energy and is heated to high intensity. For this reason, the retina can be treated either through the sclera or pupil; either way, the infrared energy will be delivered to the retinal pigment epithelium, which in turn will heat up and "cook" the adjacent retina.

CHAPTER 5

The Model Eye

1. What is the most well-known model of how the eye works as an optical system? Fill in the missing numbers in Fig. 5.1. (Answer is in Fig. 5.2.)

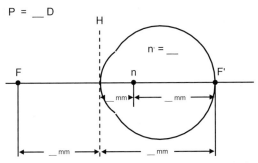

Fig. 5.1 Model of the eye as an optical system. Fill in the missing numbers.

The *reduced schematic* eye is the most well-known optical model of the eye. It is used in many optics problems because it is easier to use than more complicated models while still being accurate enough for almost all the calculations we perform. The dioptric power is +60 D, the axial length is 22.5 mm, the anterior focal length is 17 mm measured from the cornea, and the nodal point is 5.5 mm posterior to the cornea. The index of refraction is 1.33 (See Fig. 5.2).

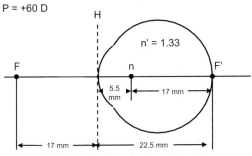

Fig. 5.2 Reduced schematic eye.

There are several other models of the eye's optical system, the most famous of which was developed by Allvar Gullstrand, who won a Nobel prize for it (the only ophthalmologist, so far, to win a Nobel prize for work in ophthalmology). His schematic eye is more complicated than the reduced schematic eye, as it has two principal planes and two nodal points. While it is useful to know the numbers from the reduced schematic eye, there is no need to memorize the numbers in the Gullstrand model; just know how it differs, in principle, from the reduced schematic eye.

2. **In the reduced schematic eye, why doesn't the nodal point coincide with the center of the lens (principal plane)?**

If the refractive index differs on two sides of a lens, the nodal point does not coincide with the principal plane. You can think of it as the higher refractive index "pulling" on the nodal point. Since the refractive index of the model eye (n = 1.33) is greater than the refractive index of air (n = 1.00), the nodal point of the eye is pulled posteriorly inside the eye (Fig 5.2).

3. **If the power of the reduced schematic model eye is +60 D, and if refraction "occurs" at the principal plane (H), why isn't the retina located 1/60 = 17 mm behind the principal plane? Why should one care about the principal plane?**

While the anterior focal point of the eye is measured from the principal plane, the posterior focal point, which coincides with the retina, is measured from the nodal point. Thus the anterior focal point is (1/60) 17 mm in front of the principal plane, while the posterior focal point is 17 mm behind the nodal point, which in turn is 5.5 mm behind the principal plane. You should care about the principal plane if you ever do ray tracing, or if you need to know the vergence of light entering the eye from a near object.

4. **What is the retinal height of a 20/200 letter (which is 8.75 cm high on a standard Snellen eye chart) when viewed at a distance of 6 m?**

The retinal height is 0.25 mm.

To calculate the retinal height of a distant image (or vice versa), we can use similar triangles (Fig. 5.3). For those of us who only have vague recollections of high school geometry, any two right triangles sharing an angle at the hypotenuse meet criteria for being "similar triangles." In this case, the ratio of the two legs of one right triangle equals the ratio of the two legs of the other right triangle. These "retinal image height" questions are exactly the type of question for which it is important to know that the nodal point is 17 mm in front of the retina.

$$\frac{\text{Object height}}{\text{Image height}} = \frac{\text{Object distance}}{\text{Image distance}}$$

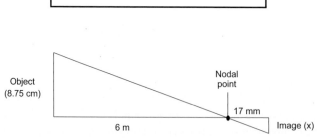

Fig. 5.3 Formula for similar triangles (and diagram of retinal height problem).

$$\frac{\text{object height (0.0875 m)}}{\text{image height (unknown)}} = \frac{\text{object distance (6 m)}}{\text{image distance (0.017 m)}}$$

$$\frac{0.0875}{X} = \frac{6}{0.017}$$

Now cross-multiply: $6 * X = (0.0875 * 0.017) = 0.00149$
Divide by 6 to solve for $X = 0.00025$ m $= 0.25$ mm

5. **Your practice was purchased by a large corporation and all the tangent screens were sold as a cost-cutting measure and to encourage the use of more lucrative visual field tests. You decide to secretly create your own tangent screen on the wall of the eye clinic. The screen will be positioned 2 m from the subject. Assuming an optic disk diameter of 1.7 mm, what size will the blind spot be on the wall?**

   The diameter is 20 cm.

   This is another similar triangle question (see previous question), but this time the object height is not known. Using similar triangles:

   $$\frac{\text{image height (1.7 mm)}}{\text{image distance (17 mm)}} = \frac{\text{object height (unknown)}}{\text{object distance (2000 mm)}}$$

   $$1.7/17 = x/2000$$
   $$17x = 2000 * 1.7$$
   $$x = (1.7 * 2000)/17$$
   $$x = 200 \text{ mm} = 20 \text{ cm}$$

6. **When silicone oil is placed in a normal phakic eye, what happens to the refractive state? Consider that the refractive index of silicone oil is 1.40, that of the crystalline lens is 1.42, and that of the vitreous is 1.33.**

   Hyperopic shift.

   In the normal phakic eye, the refractive index of the crystalline lens is 1.42 and that of the vitreous is 1.33. Since the surface with the higher refractive index is convex, the posterior surface of the lens has plus power. After a vitrectomy with silicone oil, the vitreous is replaced with silicone oil, which has a refractive index of 1.40. Therefore the posterior lens surface is still positive but substantially less so (Fig. 5.4). As a result, the typical eye will lose plus power (about 6 D).

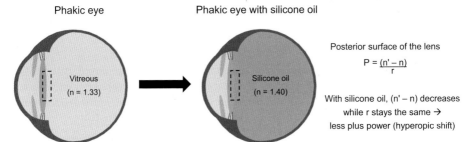

Fig. 5.4 Change in refractive state when silicone oil is placed in a phakic eye.

7. When silicone oil is inserted into an otherwise normal aphakic eye, what happens to the refractive state?

Myopic shift.

A typical aphakic eye would normally have 10–12 D of hyperopia, since the refractive contribution of the crystalline lens has been lost. When silicone oil is placed in an aphakic eye, the anterior surface of the oil has a convex shape, either in contact with the corneal endothelium (Fig. 5.5) or slightly posterior (similar end result). Since the refractive index of silicone oil (1.40) is higher than that of the aqueous (1.33) or cornea (1.37), the oil acts as a plus lens, causing a myopic shift. The extra plus power only partially compensates for the loss of the crystalline lens, so instead of having hyperopia of 10–12 D in the spectacle plane, the resulting refractive error is usually about 4–6 D of hyperopia.

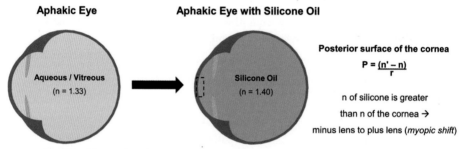

Fig. 5.5 Change in refractive state when silicone oil is placed in an aphakic eye.

8. What four factors should you consider when inserting an intraocular lens (IOL) into an eye with silicone oil?

Having silicone oil in an eye requires you to consider several factors:

1. *IOL material*: Silicone IOLs should be avoided at all costs in eyes with silicone oil (or eyes that may require silicone oil in the future) due to the irreversible adhesion of silicone oil to silicone IOLs.

2. *IOL style*: A convex-plano or meniscus-style lens (where all or most of the power of the IOL is on the anterior surface of the lens) should be selected to minimize changes in lens power after removal of silicone oil from the eye.

3. *Biometry*: Optical biometry is preferred over ultrasound, as sound travels at a different speed through silicone. If ultrasound biometry is used, corrections must be made to compensate for the slower speed of the sound waves in silicone oil. (Ultrasound machines can generally make the calculation automatically with a silicone oil setting.)

4. *IOL power calculations*: If the silicone oil will never be removed, IOL power calculations should be modified to account for the increased refractive index of silicone oil (1.40) compared to vitreous (1.33). In normal-sized eyes, about 3 D should be added to the calculated power of the IOL.

CHAPTER 6

Visual Acuity Testing

1. **How does a pinhole compensate for refractive error? How much refractive error can a pinhole correct? How can the range of efficacy of a pinhole be extended to account for higher refractive errors?**

   A pinhole decreases the blur circle created by refractive error, thereby constricting the spread of the blurred image on the retina, making the letters easier to read. A standard ophthalmic pinhole occluder can correct about 5 D of refractive error. For refractive error greater than 5 D, you can use a spherical trial lens to approximate the correction of the refractive error to within 5 D; you can then correct the remainder with a pinhole over the trial lens.

2. **What is the optimal size of a pinhole for use in the eye clinic? What happens if the pinhole is larger or smaller?**

   The optimal size is 1.2 mm.

   If the pinhole is larger, it does not shrink the blur circle as effectively. As the pinhole size is reduced, the blur circle is more effectively reduced, but diffraction begins to cause the spreading of the light. Once a certain point is reached, smaller than 1.2 mm to be exact, diffraction increases to the point that the blur circle once again begins to increase in size.

3. **What are the four types of visual acuity that can be measured? Which is the most commonly used? Which has the highest resolution?**

   1. *Minimum legible* (1 minute of arc): Smallest letters or forms that can be distinguished. This is the most common method of measuring visual acuity (e.g., Snellen, Early Treatment of Diabetic Retinopathy Study [ETDRS]).
   2. *Minimum visible* (10 seconds of arc): Minimum visual angle of an object that can be detected (even if not resolved). For example, if a person can just barely discern a copyright symbol on the bottom of the eye chart but cannot discern that it is anything more than a speck of black on a white background.
   3. *Minimum separable* (30–60 seconds of arc): The smallest visual angle at which two objects can be discriminated.
   4. *Vernier acuity* (3–5 seconds of arc): The smallest detectable amount of misalignment of two line segments. This form of visual acuity has the highest resolution.

4. **How much visual angle does an "E" on the 20/20 line subtend at 20 feet? What about an "E" on the 20/40 line? What angle would a 20/40 letter subtend at 40 feet?**

   A 20/20 "E" on a chart meant to be viewed at 20 feet is 8.75 mm tall, and each leg and space is about 1.75 mm tall. At 20 feet, the "E" subtends 5 minutes of visual angle (each leg and space subtends 1 minute of visual angle, or 1 arcmin). A 20/40 "E" subtends twice the angle, so 10 arcmin. At 40 feet, a 20/40 letter would subtend 5 arcmin (the same angle as a 20/20 letter at 20 feet, equivalent to "40/40" vision).

5. **What does logMAR stand for? What are the logMAR equivalents of 20/20, 20/40, and 20/200?**

   LogMAR stands for the *logarithm of the minimum angle of resolution.* The logMAR equivalents for 20/20, 20/40, and 20/200 are 0, 0.30, and 1.00, respectively.

EXAM PEARL

On an exam, visual acuity can be given in different formats, such as Snellen (in feet or meters), Decimal, or logMAR. It is important to know how to convert between different formats (Table 6.1). It may also be useful to commit common values to memory (in bold).

TABLE 6.1 ■ Visual Acuity Conversion Chart

Snellen (feet)	Snellen (meters)	Decimal	LogMAR = −log(1/Va)
20/20	**6/6**	**1.00**	**0.00**
20/25	6/7.5	0.80	0.10
20/32	6/9.5	0.63	0.20
20/40	**6/12**	**0.50**	**0.30**
20/50	6/15	0.40	0.40
20/63	6/19	0.32	0.50
20/80	6/24	0.25	0.60
20/100	6/30	0.20	0.70
20/125	6/38	0.16	0.80
20/160	6/48	0.125	0.90
20/200	**6/60**	**0.10**	**1.00**

6. **Your board examiner, Professor Cdhknorsvz, is a big fan of the ETDRS eye chart. Why do he and others prefer its use in large studies that use visual acuity as an outcome?**

   The ETDRS (or Ferris-Bailey) chart has several important differences from the Snellen chart (Fig. 6.1):

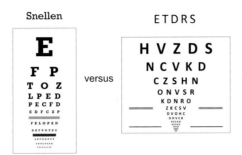

Fig. 6.1 Distance visual acuity chart comparison: Snellen versus Early Treatment of Diabetic Retinopathy Study (simulated charts to demonstrate difference).

1. All letters are Sloan optotypes; these letters (unlike those in the Snellen eye chart) were designed to have equal viewing difficulty. Professor Cdhknorsvz is particularly impressed that you are able to recite the letters, CDHKNORSVZ, in alphabetical order.
2. Each line has five letters.
3. The space between the letters is equal to the letter size on that line.
4. It is a logMAR chart; that is, the progression of optotypes is geometric, 0.1 log units (0.1 logMAR) per line.

This chart is useful in clinical research because a three-line increase (or decrease) anywhere on the chart corresponds to a doubling (or halving) of the viewing angle, making mathematical comparisons of visual acuities simpler and more accurate.

7. What is the relevance of contrast sensitivity? How is it tested?

When checking minimum legible acuity with a standard visual acuity chart, we use very high-contrast black letters on a white background. However, most visual tasks in real life are performed in lower-contrast conditions, so measuring contrast sensitivity can help determine how a patient sees outside the eye doctor's office. There are also some conditions that can have a disproportionate effect on contrast sensitivity (e.g., cataracts, optic neuritis), so a contrast sensitivity test may be a more sensitive indicator of visual dysfunction than can be determined by measuring high-contrast visual acuity.

To measure contrast sensitivity, use a room with normal background illumination (lights on). The patient should have the best refractive correction in place with undilated pupils. The patient is then presented with either sine wave gratings with progressively decreasing contrast or specially designed letter optotypes (Fig. 6.2) such as the Pelli-Robson chart.

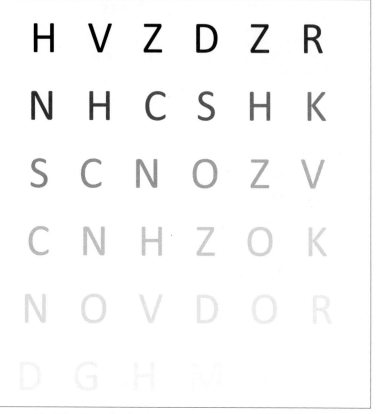

Fig. 6.2 Example of a chart used to test contrast sensitivity.

8. How is near vision quantified?

When measuring visual acuity at near, a difference of just a few inches in testing distance can change the angular resolution of the letters quite dramatically, so the testing distance must be specified. Presbyopia is also a factor when checking near acuity, so the refractive correction used during testing should be noted. Confusingly, there are several notations still in use for near visual acuity measurements:

Snellen near card: Commonly used; near visual acuity is notated in the same manner as for distance visual acuity

Jaeger eye chart: An eye chart with paragraphs of text (might be worth knowing J1 = 20/20)

M units: Reading card (again, might be worth knowing M1 = 20/50 = newspaper print)

9. How do you test visual acuity in children? Can you test vision in a child with no ability to respond?

There are several ways to test visual acuity in children. The exact testing method depends on age, development, and cooperativeness.

Coarse assessment:
- Blink/grimace to light (often the only response in a newborn)
- Optokinetic stimulus (e.g., OKN drum)
- Fix and follow

Resolution acuity:
- Preferential looking test (Teller acuity cards, Cardiff cards)
- Picture optotypes (LEA symbols) - naming or matching
- Letter optotypes (HOTV) - naming or matching

If the child does not have the ability to generate a motor response (such as eye movement), various forms of visual evoked potential (VEP) testing can be used.

10. How would you test visual acuity in an illiterate or nonverbal adult?

This may seem difficult until you realize that you see illiterate and nonverbal patients all the time: children! Any method that would work in a child would work in an illiterate or nonverbal adult. Numbers are usually a good bet when optotype acuity is needed.

11. How is visual acuity quantified when a patient with poor vision is unable to see the largest letters on a standard Snellen chart?

The most accurate way is to move the patient closer to the chart until a letter can be seen. For instance, if a patient can see a 20/400 letter at 10 feet, visual acuity is 10/400 (equivalent to 20/800). If letters cannot be perceived at any distance, testing can escalate to more coarse assessments, from counting fingers (at a certain number of feet) to hand motions to light perception (with or without projection). "No light perception" is reserved for patients who cannot detect the light from an indirect ophthalmoscope being projected directly into the eye at close range.

12. What is the definition of legal blindness in the United States and Canada?

A person is considered legally blind when their best corrected visual acuity in the better-seeing eye is *20/200 or worse*, or when the field of vision in the better-seeing eye is *20 degrees or less* in diameter. This definition is used for federal income tax status, for example. While the definition of legal blindness is uniform across the United States and Canada, requirements for the minimum vision to obtain a driver's license vary among states and provinces.

CHAPTER 7

Refraction and Optical Dispensing

1. What is the difference between axial and refractive myopia? What about between axial and refractive hyperopia?

We can define refractive error in terms of the location of the secondary focal point (i.e., the point along the optical axis where incoming parallel rays are brought to focus). In the emmetropic model eye, the focal point is on the retina (Fig. 7.1).

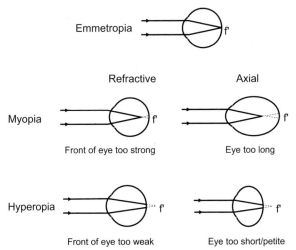

Fig. 7.1 Refractive states; emmetropia compared to refractive/axial myopia and refractive/axial hyperopia (f' is the secondary focal point of the eye).

In myopia, the focal point is in front of the retina (Fig. 7.1). In *refractive* myopia, the refractive power of the eye is too strong (more than 60 diopters [D]) while the axial length is normal. In *axial* myopia, the refractive power of the eye is normal (about 60 D) but the eye is too long.

In hyperopia, the focal point is behind the retina (Fig. 7.1). In *refractive* hyperopia, the refractive power of the eye is too weak (less than 60 D) while the axial length is normal (aphakia is the extreme example). In *axial* hyperopia, the refractive power of the eye is normal (about 60 D) but the eye is too short/petite.

2. Jai P. Rhope is a 13-year-old boy with 20/15 vision wearing +1.00 D spectacle lenses. Prior to dilation, you try reducing the hyperopic correction by 0.25 D, but this reduces visual acuity. However, during a manifest refraction, the patient continues to have 20/15 vision with +2 D of correction, only blurring when you push up to +2.25 D. On cycloplegic refraction, he requires +5 D of correction for best vision. What is the absolute hyperopia? How does that compare with the manifest hyperopia? What is meant by "facultative" hyperopia?

Absolute hyperopia = +1 D
Manifest hyperopia = +2 D
Facultative hyperopia is the amount of hyperopia controllable by the patient, who might be said to have a "facility" to exert this amount of correction.

There are five types of hyperopia (confusing, but examinable, so worth knowing; see Fig. 7.2):

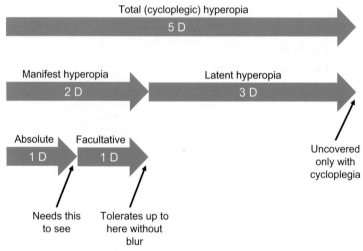

Fig. 7.2 Schematic of how the five types of hyperopia are related to each other.

1. *Cycloplegic/total hyperopia*: The total amount of hyperopia with cycloplegia = latent + manifest. In this case, +5 D.

2. *Latent hyperopia*: Tonic hyperopia, the amount of hyperopia that cannot be voluntarily relaxed, only exposed with cycloplegia. In this case there is 5 − 1 − 1 = +3 D of latent hyperopia. When latent hyperopia is large, as in this case, and a child has accommodative esotropia, it can take time for them to "relax into" stronger glasses.

3. *Manifest hyperopia*: The most plus correction the eye can accept without blurring of vision = facultative + absolute. In this case, 1 + 1 = +2 D.

4. *Facultative hyperopia*: The amount of hyperopia over and above the absolute hyperopia that can be corrected with accommodation (generally equal to accommodative amplitude). In this case, +1 D.

5. *Absolute hyperopia*: The least amount of plus correction required for clear vision at distance. Not to be confused with total hyperopia. In this case, +1 D.

We generally prescribe somewhere between the absolute hyperopia and the manifest hyperopia, depending on the clinical scenario and patient preference, but will build up to the latent hyperopia when needed in cases of accommodative esotropia or persistent asthenopia.

3. **Ms. Minh U. Shah requires +2 D to see at distance. The most she can tolerate is +4.5 D. Cycloplegic refraction is +5 D. What are the absolute, manifest, facultative, latent, and total hyperopia?**

As per the definitions just described (Fig. 7.3):

Absolute = minimum needed to see = +2 D

Manifest = maximum can accept and see clearly = +4.5 D

Facultative = manifest − absolute = 4.5 − 2 = +2.5 D

Latent = cycloplegic − manifest = 5 − 4.5 = +0.5 D

Total = cycloplegic = +5 D

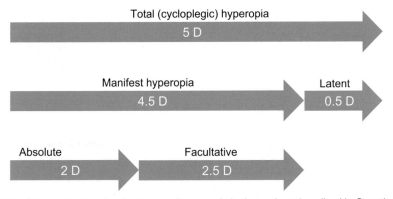

Fig. 7.3 Schematic showing five types of hyperopia in the patient described in Question 3.

4. **Reg Metogenus returns to your office complaining of blurry vision in the left eye just 4 months after you performed a refraction. On examination, you find a change in refractive error from +1.00 D to −2.00 D in the left eye only. What is this called? What are some possible causes?**

This is called *acquired myopia* (or a *myopic shift*). The cause can be divided into things that make the eye too *long* (axial) or too *strong* (refractive) (Table 7.1). On further questioning, the patient recalls that since he last saw you, he had a retinal detachment with a scleral buckle on the left. Just a 1-mm increase in axial length from the buckle can cause a 3 D myopic shift.

TABLE 7.1 ■ Causes of Acquired Myopia

Things that increase axial length (eye too long)

Pathologic
  Congenital glaucoma
  Posterior staphyloma
  Idiopathic progressive myopia
Iatrogenic
  Scleral buckle

Things that increase refractive error (eye too strong)

Increased corneal curvature
  Keratoconus
Increased lens power (increased curvature or refractive index)
  Cataract (nuclear sclerosis)
  Diabetes
  Lenticonus
Anterior lens shift (increased effective power)
  Traumatic anterior lens dislocation
  Ciliary muscle spasm
  Increased ciliary muscle tone (pregnancy, certain drugs)
  Ciliochoriodal effusion

5. **Caesar Free, a 48-year-old previously emmetropic man with epilepsy, presents to your office complaining of sudden onset of blurry vision and mild eye pain in both eyes. Refraction reveals 4.5 D of myopia in each eye. What are two possible reasons for the sudden, symmetric myopia?**

> There are a few possibilities. One is the new onset of diabetes, which can cause acquired myopia due to a change in the refractive index of the crystalline lens (and increased curvature in some cases).
>
> Another possibility could be the medication being used to control his seizures. Topiramate (Topomax) has been reported to cause sudden myopia and increased intraocular pressure resulting from idiosyncratic ciliochoroidal effusion occurring in rare cases. Two mechanisms for the myopia are likely: (1) forward displacement of the iris–lens diaphragm (increased effective plus power; see Chapter 8, Lens Effectivity and Vertex Distance) and (2) relaxation of zonular tension and subsequent increased convexity of the crystalline lens (increased power). Myopia (and acute glaucoma, which also may occur if the lens and iris shift far enough forward) does not typically respond to peripheral iridectomy due to the complete abutment of the lens against the iris, but it will respond to administration of cycloplegic drops (such as atropine).

6. **What is the differential diagnosis of acquired hyperopia (hyperopic shift)?**

> Like myopia, hyperopia can be due to axial or refractive changes. In hyperopia, the eye becomes too *petite* (axial) or too *weak* (refractive) (Table 7.2).

TABLE 7.2 ■ **Causes of Acquired Hyperopia**

Things that decrease axial length (eye is too petite)

Decrease in *actual* axial length
Orbital mass with pressure on posterior globe
Decrease in *effective* axial length
Central serous retinopathy
Choroidal tumor (e.g., choroidal melanoma)

Things that decrease refractive error (eye is too weak)

Decreased corneal curvature
Orthokeratology (ortho-K)
Decreased lens power
Aphakia
Complete lens dislocation
Posterior lens shift (loss of effective lens power)
Posterior lens dislocation
Weak accommodation (e.g., third nerve palsy, Adie's tonic pupil, concussion, certain drugs)

7. Name a retinal cause of acquired astigmatism.

Trick question. Astigmatism *cannot* be caused by retinal disease, only by external, corneal, or lenticular factors.

8. Okay, smarty pants, what are some *nonretinal* causes of acquired astigmatism?

Acquired astigmatism is generally due to external, corneal, or lenticular causes (Table 7.3).

TABLE 7.3 ■ **Causes of Acquired Astigmatism**

Things that cause astigmatism

External causes
Masses (e.g., dermoid cyst, lid tumor, chalazion)
Ptosis
Corneal causes
Keratoconus
Pellucid marginal degeneration
Pterygium
Lenticular causes
Ciliary body tumor
Lenticonus
Ectopia lentis
Lens coloboma

9. **Red Phlagg, a 78-year-old man, presents with blurry vision in his left eye. On examination, visual acuity is 20/20 OD and 20/80 OS. He was plano OU last year, and now you find a refraction of plano OD and –1.00 +5.00 × 60 in the left eye, giving him visual acuity of 20/25 OS. On slit lamp exam, the corneas appear normal. Dilated fundus examination is normal. What should you be concerned about?**

Ciliary body tumor.

The marked shift in astigmatism with no obvious cause is classic for a problem in the area of the ciliary body. The next step would be to repeat the fundus examination, this time with scleral depression. In some cases, transillumination of the globe can be helpful. The definitive evaluation would be an ultrasound biomicroscopy (UBM) to check for a ciliary body mass. Acquired lenticular astigmatism is a red flag for a ciliary body tumor, such as a melanoma. These are uncommon but life-threatening, so important to think about on an exam (and in real life too!).

EXAM PEARL

Watch for acquired refractive error as a sign of a potentially vision- or life-threatening disease. Important examples include:

- Progressive myopia in an infant; *congenital glaucoma*
- Acquired hyperopia; *choroidal tumor (e.g., choroidal melanoma) or orbital tumor (e.g., rhabdomyosarcoma, orbital metastasis)*
- Unexplained new unilateral astigmatism; *ciliary body tumor*

10. **Ankoor Theman is a 27-year-old engineering prodigy and budding physician scientist with a refraction of −8.00 sphere in both eyes. He is concerned about the weight and appearance of his glasses. What interventions might you offer?**

High minus glasses have thick edges and minify the eyes. There are several options that may help:

1. *Check refraction*: Make sure all the minus is needed. Re-refract carefully and consider a cycloplegic refraction.

2. *Get rid of glasses:* Contact lenses, refractive surgery, or a phakic intraocular lens (IOL) (younger patients) or refractive lens exchange (older patients) may be options.

3. *Adjust the lenses:*
   - Use high-index material (decreases the thickness of lenses; see explanation in Question 13)
   - Smaller frames (minus lenses get thicker at the edges)
   - Bevel and polish the edges of the lens (hides thickened edges)
   - Flatten the base curve (since most lenses have plus power on the front, extra minus must be ground into the rear of the lens to compensate; a flatter base curve reduces the need to grind in as much extra minus and thereby reduces the perceived thickness)

11. **Captain Hawkeye, a 27-year-old army surgeon whom you have painstakingly refracted, returns complaining of trouble with her distance vision, especially at**

night. You repeat your refraction and obtain exactly the same results. What are some probable causes of the patient's complaints?

She likely has *night myopia*. Several factors may contribute:

1. *Spherical aberration*: When the pupil dilates at night, the periphery of the lens is exposed allowing light rays to pass through the peripheral lens; these rays are refracted more strongly. "Too strong" = more myopia.

2. *Chromatic aberration*: In lower light levels, spectral sensitivity shifts to shorter (blue) wavelengths (Purkinje shift) that are refracted more strongly than longer wavelengths, producing a wavelength-determined myopia.

3. *Lack of an accommodative target*: Patients may look at pinpoints of light and, with no letters to validate the accuracy of accommodation, overaccommodate. Like a deer in headlights.

4. *Finite length of refractive lane*: A refraction lane is 20 feet (6 meters), which means that patients are $1/6$ D $= 0.167$ D undercorrected for infinity. Road signs are usually read from much more than 20 feet away.

Night myopia can generally be alleviated by adding another -0.25 D to the prescription. For patients in the prepresbyopic range who are symptomatic, this may necessitate separate "night driving" glasses to avoid creating problems with increased accommodative demand at near.

12. **Mr. A. Faykia detests his +15 D glasses, strongly preferring contact lenses to the point of risking injury to his eyes from overwear. Describe some problems with high-plus-powered spectacles that might discourage him from going without contact lenses.**

1. *Ring scotoma*: Due to the prismatic effect of the lenses, there is a ring scotoma that causes a "Jack-in-the-box" phenomenon (things seem to appear out of nowhere).

2. *Pincushion distortion*: The periphery of an image is magnified more than the center (contrast with the "barrel distortion" of high minus lenses).

3. *Excessive magnification*: While this may not bother the patient in terms of what he can see, it may have a negative cosmetic effect, both because the lenses look like the bottoms of a Coke bottle, and because the eyes look especially large.

4. *Weight*: Aphakic spectacles can be quite heavy (several times heavier than low-power spectacles).

5. *Cost*: Expensive (hundreds of dollars extra).

13. **What is the main advantage of high-index lenses? Why might a patient dislike high-index lenses?**

High-index lenses allow for the lenses to be thinner (for the same power). If we refer to the formula for the power of a spherical surface, $P = (n' - n)/r$ (see Chapter 2, Vergence, Lenses, Objects, and Images), we can see that if n' is higher (higher refractive index), then $(n' - n)$ is larger. This allows for r to be larger (the radius of curvature is not as steep) while still yielding the same power. Since a high-index minus lens will be less curved, it will not be as thick at the edges and it will not be as heavy. High-index lenses provide a particular advantage for high-power lenses.

The two main disadvantages of high-index lenses are that they may have more chromatic aberration (lower Abbe number), and the area of the lens giving the clearest vision, the "sweet spot," tends to be smaller than with ordinary plastic lenses. They are also more expensive.

14. **You typically retinoscope at a working distance of 67 cm from the patient, but you had an accident recently (involving a heavy prism bar and a recalcitrant child). As a result, you temporarily cannot extend your arms as far, and you must perform retinoscopy at 50 cm. How should you modify the value obtained at neutralization to obtain the refraction at infinity before and after the accident? You decide to replace your arms with robotic arm extensions (with built-in retinoscope) and you now refract at 1 m. How will this change your refraction?**

Before your accident, you subtracted 1.50 D (i.e., you modified the value obtained at neutralization by 1.50 D in the minus direction).
After the accident, you should subtract 2.00 D.
With robotic arms, subtract only 1.00 D.

At neutralization, the patient's eye is in focus at the peephole of the retinoscope (i.e., the far point of the patient's eye is at the peephole of your retinoscope), which was 0.67 m (before the accident) and is now 0.50 m (after the accident). To move the far point of the eye to infinity, you need to take the reciprocal of your working distance and subtract this from the values you obtained at your working distance. So, $1/0.67$ m $= 1.50$ D was subtracted from the refraction obtained at neutralization before the accident and $1/0.50$ m $= 2.00$ D should be subtracted after the accident. If you opt for the cool robotic arm extensions, you are now 1 m away, so $1/1$ m $= 1.00$ D should be subtracted to obtain the refraction at infinity. (The robotic arms have also turned out to be very helpful at keeping recalcitrant children in check.)

15. **A 25-year-old accountant presents to your clinic for refraction. He had early bilateral congenital cataract extractions in infancy, followed by corneal transplants for keratoconus (complicated by herpes simplex virus keratitis). One pupil is 9 mm and irregular, the other is 4 mm and irregular. Uncorrected visual acuity is 20/400 OU, but it improves to a brisk 20/30 in each eye through a pinhole. The retinotopic reflex is very poor. What do you do now?**

There are several things that may help with a challenging retinoscopy:
1. Concentrate as much as possible on the central portion of the retinoscopic reflex.
2. Use a retinoscope with a bright halogen light source.
3. Move closer (remember to adjust for your closer working distance).
4. Try an autorefractor (unfortunately, it may be inaccurate, or the instrument might simply refuse to cooperate with such a difficult eye).
5. Put your best estimate of the refraction in the phoropter (or previous glasses or refraction if available) and subjectively refine. You may need to use large (1.00 D) increments in sphere and a high-power Jackson cross cylinder, as smaller increments may not produce a discernible change when visual acuity is poor.

6. Place a rigid trial contact lens and perform an overrefraction. The contact lens will reduce irregular astigmatism caused by the diseased corneal surface.
7. Consider a stenopeic slit refraction (see next question).

16. Describe a stenopeic slit and how to use it in refraction. Are there any drawbacks? What is the refraction if a patient reports best visual acuity with +10.00 D (stenopeic slit at 165 degrees) and +6.00 (stenopeic slit at 75 degrees)?

A stenopeic slit is an elongated pinhole that can help determine *subjective* astigmatic refractive error, especially when the retinoscopic reflex is poor (e.g., irregular astigmatism, small pupils, media opacities). It is not commonly used in practice but remains commonly used on exams. To use a stenopeic slit (in theory):
1. Before putting the slit in place, use spheres to put the midpoint of the conoid of Sturm close to the retina (i.e., get the best preliminary focus).
2. Put the slit in place and rotate until the patient reports the best acuity. If there is no change as the slit is rotated, you may have placed the circle of least confusion precisely on the retina in Step 1; change the sphere slightly and try again.
3. Add plus or minus sphere to sharpen the image (position 1). This sphere moves the focal line that is perpendicular to the slit onto the retina. Note the total amount of sphere.
4. Rotate the slit 90 degrees (position 2) and add plus or minus sphere (you have no way of knowing which it will be) until the sharpest image is obtained.
5. Record the two values on a power cross and convert to the refraction. Note that the output of the stenopeic slit is a *power* cross, not an *axis* cross.

An important drawback of stenopeic slit refraction (other than the fact that no one uses it) is that the slit must be perfectly centered in the pupil or the patient will notice little or no change in the image as the slit is rotated. This position can be difficult to maintain, even for a cooperative patient. If a patient notes the best vision with +10 D (slit at 165 degrees) and +6 D (slit at 75 degrees), the corrective lens would be +10.00 −4.00 × 165 (or +6.00 +4.00 × 75; See Chapter 10, Cylinders, Crosses, and Spherocylindrical Notation). This should be refined subjectively.

17. What is an "error lens" and why is it a useful concept?

When an eye is myopic, it can be thought of as "too strong" because light rays are brought into focus in front of the retina. One way to simulate an eye that is too strong is to insert extra plus power in the eye. That is, if Dr. West were emmetropic and Dr. Hunter surgically inserted a +10 D iris claw anterior chamber IOL in her eye (as a birthday present) without disturbing her natural lens, she would end up as a myope requiring slightly less than −10 D of contact lens correction to see clearly at distance. The +10 D surgically implanted IOL can be considered an "error lens" (in more ways than one). Similarly, the error lens in a hyperopic person has minus power. The error lens concept is especially useful when calculating magnification caused by the correction of ametropia.

18. **Why do patients respond that things look "smaller" when they are "overminused" during a refraction?**

Glasses can combine with the error lens of the eye to form a Galilean telescope (see Chapter 17, Instruments). Too much minus in the trial frame or phoropter effectively forms the eyepiece of a Galilean telescope, and the extra plus power in the eye (the error lens) forms the objective. The patient's retina is thus looking through a backward Galilean telescope, and the letters are minified.

19. **What is iseikonia? What is aniseikonia and what causes it?**

Iseikonia is when there is no difference in perceived image size between the two eyes.

Aniseikonia is when there is a difference in perceived image size between eyes. Most normal adults can tolerate a 6–8% difference in image size, and children can tolerate even more. Aniseikonia is most commonly caused by the correction of unequal refractive errors (e.g., monocular aphakia) but can also be found with retinal problems and occipital lobe lesions. A handy rule of thumb for spectacle correction is that each diopter changes the retinal image size by about 2% (plus lenses magnify, minus lenses minify), so most adults can tolerate about 3–4 D of difference in glasses (kids can tolerate much more).

20. **What is anisometropia?**

Anisometropia is a difference in refractive error between the two eyes. For children, anisometropia is important because it can cause amblyopia. In adults, anisometropia is important because it can cause aniseikonia and is most likely to be problematic if the refraction of the eye changes (e.g., after cataract surgery). The popular definition of clinically significant anisometropia (~3–4 D of spherical difference between the eyes) is good to know but not a hard rule. Many factors determine the amount of anisometropia a given patient can tolerate, such as the type of anisometropia, duration, patient age, binocularity and fusional potential, and the type of correction (spectacles versus contact lenses).

21. **What is Knapp's rule? Does it apply to axial or refractive myopia or both? Should it be used clinically to treat aniseikonia in a patient with unilateral high myopia?**

Knapp's rule states that the proper corrective lens placed at the anterior focal point of an eye will produce retinal images of the same size no matter what amount of *axial* ametropia exists. Two problems prevent this from being strictly applied in clinical practice: ametropia is almost never purely axial, and it is impractical to set a vertex distance of 17 mm for spectacle correction (typical vertex distance is 12 mm). Furthermore, the retina in the myopic eye of a patient with unilateral high myopia is stretched; this increase in the separation of photoreceptors can cause confounding changes in effective magnification.

22. **Trey Dur-Jo is a 69-year-old grocer who underwent surgery for a left unilateral traumatic cataract. He says that his surgeon was very proud of her IOL calculations and toric IOL implantation despite the complexity of his case, as he is now**

plano in that eye. Unfortunately, he has been having headaches and dizziness since the surgery. He is wearing glasses of −6 D OD and plano OS.

(a) What is the likely cause of his symptoms and what can you do to help?

The problem is probably arising from anisometropia. Most adults can only tolerate about 3–4 D of anisometropia while wearing glasses (6–8% aniseikonia). To help, you have a few options:

    i. IOL exchange in the left eye (to within 3 D of the other eye, likely aim for around −3 D)

    ii. Clear lens extraction in the right eye (with refractive goal between plano and −3 D)

    iii. Contact lenses or refractive surgery

(b) Would anything be different if Trey were a 6-year-old wearing −6 D OD and plano OS after unilateral cataract surgery?

Yes!

Kids can tolerate much higher amounts of anisometropia (the younger they are, the more they can tolerate), so it is unlikely that he would be symptomatic. For treatment, if needed, clear lens extraction is usually not performed in children because of the additional downside of loss of accommodation.

CHAPTER 8

Lens Effectivity and Vertex Distance

1. What is vertex distance and why is it important?

Vertex distance is the distance from the cornea to the back surface of a corrective lens (usually around 12 mm in glasses and 0 mm in contacts). It matters because *lens effectivity changes with vertex distance.* This means that, as vertex distance changes (e.g., changing from glasses to contact lenses or back), the power of the optical correction must be adjusted to maintain the same effective power.

The amount of change in lens effectivity varies in proportion to the power of the lens, so vertex distance is only important with higher-power spectacles (> 5 diopters [D]). Vertex distance also influences *magnification* caused by lenses and *distortion* caused by astigmatic correction.

2. How do you measure vertex distance?

Vertex distance is most accurately measured with a vertex distance measuring device such as a *distometer* (also known as a *vertexometer*). The distometer measures the distance from the back of the lens to the surface of the *closed* eyelid. The scale takes the average thickness of the eyelid (2 mm) into account, and the vertex distance is read directly from the scale on the instrument. It is also possible to simply view the patient in profile, hold a ruler next to the glasses, and estimate the distance. The phoropter has a mirror and scale on the side that may be used to measure vertex distance. The distance can be adjusted on the phoropter by adjusting the forehead rest using the knob in the center of the instrument.

3. What is the far point of the eye? Where are the far points for someone who has emmetropia, hyperopia, and myopia?

The *far point* is the point of focus of the eye with accommodation completely relaxed (measured from the cornea). A person with emmetropia can see clearly at distance, so the far point is at infinity. For a person with hyperopia, the far point is behind the cornea. For someone with myopia, the far point is in front of the cornea. To calculate the location of the far point, take the reciprocal of the refractive error: 1/refractive error (in diopters) = distance of the far point from the cornea (in meters).

4. Why would a man with hyperopia slide his glasses down his nose? What happens if a woman with myopia moves her glasses down her nose?

Moving a lens, either plus or minus, away from the eye gives it more effective plus power (i.e., a plus lens gets *more* effective plus power and a minus lens gets *less* effective minus power). To correct any refractive error with glasses, one must find a lens with a secondary focal point that coincides with the far point of the eye. This is so that light from infinity is focused at the far point of the eye, meaning that a distance target is in focus with accommodation completely relaxed.

In a patient with hyperopia, the far point is behind the eye. If the plus lens is too weak (i.e., the hyperopia is undercorrected), the focal point of the lens is behind the far point of the eye. Moving the lens forward moves the focal point of the lens closer to the far point of the eye (the lens effectively has more plus power). Thus, the patient with hyperopia in this example is either undercorrected for distance or would like more plus power to see clearly at near.

In a patient with myopia, the far point is in front of the eye. Moving the minus lens forward moves the focal point of the lens in front of the far point of the eye (the lens again has more plus power → *less* minus power). Why would a person with myopia slide her glasses down her nose if it makes the glasses less powerful? The extra plus power may be useful for near work, but it will cause undercorrection for distance. If the reading material is held close to the focal point of a plus lens, the rules change a bit, but we will save that topic for our next book, *I've Got Nothing Else to Do but Study Optics.*

5. **An entrepreneur is fully corrected with –10.00 D spectacles at a vertex distance of 10 mm. He is beta-testing a new augmented-reality device that can accommodate spectacle lenses but with an unfortunate limitation of requiring a 20-mm vertex distance.**

    (a) **What correction will be needed if the spectacles are positioned 20 mm away from the eye?**

        –11.0 D.

        This is a standard vertex distance problem that is very common on exams. As with many optics questions, you may find it helpful to draw a diagram. In this case, draw the eye and the lens (Fig. 8.1, *top*).

        Step 1: Find the far point of the eye (myopia → far point is *in front of* the eye). The far point is 1/10 D = 0.1 m = 100 mm in front of the lens, or 110 mm in front of the eye (it may help to convert from m to mm for these calculations). Now that you know the location of the far point, you can forget about where the spectacles used to be (that number will only confuse you). To emphasize this point, we redraw the diagram (Fig. 8.1, *middle*).

        Step 2: Insert the new lens and calculate the distance from the new lens to the far point of the eye (Fig. 8.1, *bottom*). The new spectacle plane is 20 mm in front of the eye, and so it is (110 – 20) = 90 mm from the far point.

        Step 3: Take a reciprocal of the distance of the new lens from the far point. The required power is (1/0.090 m) = –11.1 D. The closest power available is –11.0 D.

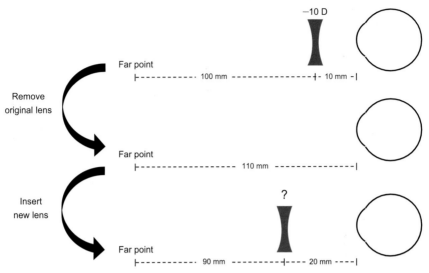

Fig. 8.1 Vertex distance diagram for myopia. Calculate the far point by taking the reciprocal of lens power, then remove the lens to show the distance of the far point from the cornea, and finally, insert the new lens and calculate the power, P = 1/distance of new lens to far point.

To review, the three steps are:

1. Take a reciprocal and add or subtract vertex distance to find the far point of the eye relative to the cornea.
2. Add or subtract to find the distance of the new lens to the far point.
3. Take a reciprocal of the new distance (in m) to get a new power (in diopters).

(b) **The engineers come up with a new beta device to address the problem; this time it requires that the spectacle lenses be positioned at a 5-mm vertex distance. What power is needed now?**

−9.5 D.

(110 − 5 = 105 mm; 1/0.105 m = 9.5 D).

(c) **The engineers respond to the unreasonable demands of a normal vertex distance of 12 mm and state that only contact lens users can wear the device. What power soft contact lens will probably be required?**

−9.0 D.

(1/0.110 m = 9.1 D; closest power available is − 9.0 D).

(d) **The next innovation is a giant helmet device that holds lenses 10 cm away from the eye. What power lens would be needed in this case?**

−100 D.

(110 − 100 = 10 mm; 1/0.010 m = 100 D).

6. **What if the patient in the previous problem had +10.00 D hyperopia with the same vertex distance of 10 mm? Determine the lens power required for the same vertex distances, namely:**

   (a) **20 mm**

   (b) **5 mm**

   (c) **Contact lens**

   (d) **10 cm**

   In this case, the far point is $1/10 = 0.1$ m $= 100$ mm *behind* the spectacles, or $(100 - 10) = 90$ mm behind the cornea (Fig. 8.2).

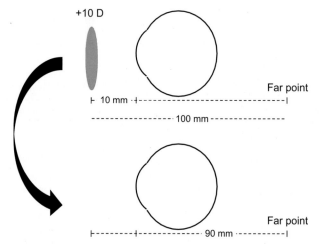

+10 D

⊢ 10 mm ⊦------------------------------- Far point
---------------- 100 mm ----------------

Far point
⊢--------⊦------------ 90 mm ----------⊣

Fig. 8.2   Vertex distance diagram for a patient with hyperopia. Calculate the far point by taking the reciprocal of lens power, then remove the lens to show the distance of the far point from the cornea, and finally, insert the new lens and calculate the power, P = 1/distance of new lens to far point.

   (a) **+9.0 D.** A lens 20 mm in front of the eye is $(90 + 20) = 110$ mm away from the far point, so the power required is $(1/0.110$ m$) = +9.1$ D, with +9.0 being the closest power available.
   (b) **+10.5 D.** $(90 + 5) = 95$ mm. $(1/0.095) = +10.5$ D.
   (c) **+11.0 D.** $(1/0.090) = +11.1$ D, with 11.0 D being the closest power available.
   (d) **+5.25 D.** $(100 + 90) = 190$ mm. $(1/0.19$ m$) = +5.25$ D. Contrast this with the myopic situation where the required power increases to -100 D.

7. **What can happen to best-corrected distance visual acuity measurement when a person with high myopia goes from glasses to contact lenses (or has refractive surgery)? Why? What about a person with high hyperopia?**

   Measured visual acuity may appear to improve for a patient with high myopia switching to contact lenses.

   Measured visual acuity may appear to worsen for a patient with high hyperopia switching to contact lenses.

A person with myopia in glasses effectively has a reverse Galilean telescope, which causes minification of the image. Moving the point of correction of a patient with myopia from the spectacle plane to the corneal plane reduces the required minus power and gives a corresponding increase in the magnification of the image, such that best-corrected visual acuity may improve.

Conversely, best-corrected visual acuity may decline slightly when hyperopic correction is moved from the spectacle plane to the corneal plane. This is because a person with hyperopia in glasses effectively has magnification from a Galilean telescope, so the loss of the telescope effect causes a loss of magnification and a corresponding worsening of best-corrected visual acuity.

8. **During a planned 3-hour boat tour, some rough weather has stranded you and your shipmates on a small desert island. The group includes the skipper, with –5 D spectacle-corrected myopia; his only crew member, Gilligan; and a professor of optics, known simply as "the professor." Unfortunately, Gilligan dropped the skipper's glasses (which had an 11-mm vertex distance) down the opening of an active volcano. There is no prospect of returning the group to safety without replacing the skipper's glasses, but the only lens available is a –55 D Hruby lens, which the professor happens to have on hand.**

   (a) **How many centimeters from the eye should the skipper hold the lens to fully correct the refractive error?**

   19.3 cm.

   First, locate the far point. The far point is 211 mm in front of the eye (Fig. 8.3). The new lens has a power of –55 D, which means its focal point is $(1/55) = 0.018$ m or 18 mm away from the lens. To correct the refractive error, the focal point of the lens should coincide with the far point of the eye. Therefore, it should be 18 mm away from the far point, or $(211 - 18) = 193$ mm (19.3 cm) in front of the eye.

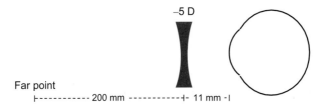

   Fig. 8.3 Far point of the stranded skipper described in Question 8.

   (b) **Would the skipper be able to read the 20/20 line with this correction? Why or why not?**

   No.

   The problem is magnification. This configuration turns the combination of the eye and its corrective lens into a reverse Galilean telescope, which significantly minifies the image. The eyepiece is approximately +5 D (the error lens of the myopic eye) and the objective lens is −55 D. The resulting magnification is (5/55) ≅ 0.1×. Since the image would be 10× smaller, he would likely only be able to read about 20/200 (assuming an otherwise normal eye). Similarly, patients with very high myopia who are properly corrected may not be able to read 20/20 through their spectacle lenses, even in the absence of other pathology.

CHAPTER 9

Accommodation, Presbyopia, and Bifocals

1. What is accommodation? How do you describe a patient's ability to accommodate?

Accommodation is the process by which an eye increases its total dioptric power by increasing the convexity of the lens through ciliary muscle contraction. For simplicity, assume that this additional plus power is acting at the cornea.

The *amplitude of accommodation* is the maximum number of diopters (D) that the eye can accommodate (expressed in D). It is related to the physical ability of the lens of the eye to change shape during accommodation.

The *range of accommodation* is the linear distance over which a patient can accommodate and maintain clear vision (expressed as two locations between which the patient can see clearly). The range of acommodation is determined by the patient's amplitude of accommodation and underlying refractive error.

2. What is the near point of the eye? Where are the near points for someone who is emmetropic, hyperopic, and myopic?

The *near point* is the point of focus of the eye with accommodation maximally active (measured from the cornea). Compare this to the *far point*, which is the point of focus when accommodation is fully relaxed (see Chapter 8, Lens Effectivity and Vertex Distance). Unlike the far point, the location of the near point relative to the cornea cannot be determined from the refractive error of the eye alone, since it also depends on the accommodative amplitude.

3. How do you measure accommodative amplitude?

Accommodative amplitude can be quantified in two ways. For both methods, one eye is tested at a time and the patient should be in best distance correction.

(1) *Prince rule or Royal Air Force (RAF) rule*: The Prince and RAF rules are rulers scaled in both diopters and centimeters; the Prince rule attaches to the phoropter while the RAF rule is used in free space. Position the target on the rule at a distance that allows the patient to see the letters clearly. Slowly move the target closer to the eye while encouraging the patient to keep it in focus. Record the point (in D) at which the patient first reports that the target is just beginning to blur.

If a patient has trouble accommodating even to the end of the RAF or Prince rule (1 D), it is necessary to provide an add prior to measuring the amplitude of accommodation. For example, if you start with a +3 add, place the target at +3 on the rule. If the image begins to blur at +4 (25 cm), then the patient has a 1 D amplitude of accommodation.

(2) *Method of spheres*: In this case, ask the patient to focus on a reading target (e.g., at 40 cm). Slowly add minus sphere while encouraging the patient to keep the target in focus. Record the amount of minus sphere at which the target blurs. Then add progressively stronger plus sphere until the target blurs. The difference in power between the two lenses is the accommodative amplitude.

4. How much accommodation is normal?

Humans lose accommodative amplitude with age. There are several tables and formulas to calculate the expected accommodative amplitude, such as Donder's Table (Table 9.1).

TABLE 9.1 ■ Donder's Table for Estimation of Accommodative Amplitude by Age

Age (years)	20	24	28	32	36	40	44	48	52	56	60	64	68
Accommodation* (D)	11	10	9	8	7	6	4.5	3	2.5	2	1.5	1	0.5

*The key reference points for this table include the following: A 40-year-old has about 6 D and a 48-year-old has 3 D, with a gain of 1 D for every 4 years younger than 40, and a loss of 0.5 D for every 4 years older than 48.

5. **Phil Attly, a 48-year-old hobbyist, complains of eye strain after a long session of practicing philately. His current prescription is −0.50 D sphere in both eyes, which the patient wears full time. You astutely diagnose presbyopia and recommend bifocals.**

   (a) **How do you determine the best add to alleviate Phil's symptoms?**

   The formal procedure for prescribing bifocals includes the following steps:
   - Determine the preferred working distance and convert to diopters (this is the required amount of accommodation).
   - Measure the accommodative amplitude.
   - Divide the accommodative amplitude in half (we would not expect a person to exert their full accommodative amplitude for near work, but most people are fine exerting about half).
   - Subtract half the accommodative amplitude from the required accommodation.

   (b) **You learn that Mr. Attly prefers to view stamps (without magnification) at a distance of 33 cm. You measure accommodative amplitude and discover it is exactly on target for age 48, at 3 D. What power of bifocal would you prescribe? What about single vision reading glasses?**

   Give +1.50 D bifocal, +1.00 D single vision reading glasses

   To view stamps at a distance of 33 cm requires 3 D of accommodation. Phil has 3 D of accommodative amplitude but would be uncomfortable maximally accommodating for hours at a time, so we divide 3 D in half to give 1.5 D. You would then prescribe a bifocal add of 3 − 1.50 = 1.50 D.

Alternatively, Phil could remove the −0.50 glasses for near work. This would give him an extra 0.50 D of power (the myopic "error lens"), but since he needs 1.50 D of extra power to read comfortably, he would still benefit from +1.00 D single vision reading glasses.

(c) **Do you always need to check accommodative amplitude before prescribing bifocals or reading glasses? When is it important to measure accommodative amplitude?**

Realistically, you are not going to measure accommodative amplitude in every patient, so it is acceptable to estimate accommodative amplitude and use the steps from part **(a)** when selecting a bifocal add. However, if Phil was only 32 years old yet symptomatic from prolonged near work, you might want to measure accommodative amplitude to see if it is lower than expected for his age (not to mention performing a cycloplegic refraction to check for latent hyperopia). Other circumstances for measuring accommodative amplitude include when a patient is not happy with new reading glasses or if there is concern about accommodative insufficiency from drugs, trauma, or other disease.

Even more realistically, when the symptoms are minimal but typical of presbyopia, it is okay to start a patient off with a +1.25 D add as a first step and build up in increments over years as accommodation inevitably declines. Just do not tell anybody we said that.

6. **What are progressive addition bifocal lenses and how might you counsel a potential progressive addition lens wearer?**

Progressive addition lenses (PALs) have a channel of progressively higher (plus) dioptric power on the front of the lens, effectively creating a variable-focus bifocal. While there is no line to bother the cosmetically conscious, there can be marked irregular peripheral astigmatism. This can be annoying, especially in higher-power PALs. Patients who have already worn traditional bifocals have the greatest difficulty accepting the distortion of a PAL. Those newly diagnosed with presbyopia requiring a low-power add are most likely to do well with PALs.

7. **During an office visit you find that an 18-month-old child continues to accommodate after receiving the typical dilation cocktail. You ask for repeat dilation and, after an hour, you are pleased to see that the cycloplegia appears to be complete. Later that day, the mother calls stating that the child has developed a fever and is very fussy. Her face seems red. What do you think might be happening and how should you proceed?**

The signs are concerning for *anticholinergic toxicity*. The child may have been given several drops of atropine or higher concentrations of cyclopentolate. This is a toxic reaction (an anticholinergic overdose), not an idiosyncratic or allergic reaction. Since it is possible that this is a severe reaction, you should bring the patient in or send her to a nearby emergency room for prompt evaluation. If there is a significant overdose, supportive therapy (i.e., sponge baths for fever, catheterization for urinary retention, oxygen for mild respiratory depression) is usually enough, but severe reactions may require treatment with intravenous physostigmine or intubation for respiratory depression. This mnemonic may help you remember the signs and symptoms of atropine toxicity (i.e., anticholinergic toxicity):

- *Hot as a hare*: increased body temperature
- *Blind as a bat*: dilated pupils and impaired accommodation
- *Dry as a bone*: dry mouth, dry skin, and dry eyes
- *Red as a beet*: flushed face, lightheadedness, and fainting
- *Mad as a hatter*: confusion, anxiety, rapid heart rate, and headache

Facial flushing in the absence of fever may also occur after the administration of even a single drop of atropine. This is not necessarily a sign of an overdose, but when patients show this reaction, they should not receive further atropine drops.

8. Do the same effects occur with phenylephrine?

No.

Phenylephrine cannot cause anticholinergic toxicity; it has no cycloplegic effect. It is a sympathomimetic agent used for pupillary dilation alone. Excessive amounts of phenylephrine *can* cause hypertension as well as reflex bradycardia.

9. A child with emmetropia named Reese Iprocal has an accommodative amplitude of 20 D. What is the near point? What is the range of accommodation?

The near point is 5 cm. The range of accommodation is infinity to 5 cm.

To calculate the near point, calculate the maximum dioptric power and take the reciprocal: (refractive error + accommodative amplitude) = 0 + 20 = 20 D, near point: 1/20 D = 0.05 m = 5 cm (Fig. 9.1). To calculate the range of accommodation, calculate the far and near points. For a patient with emmetropia, the far point is at infinity and the near point is = 1/accommodative amplitude = 5 cm (Fig. 9.1).

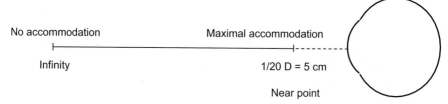

No accommodation   Maximal accommodation

Infinity   1/20 D = 5 cm

Near point

Fig. 9.1   Reese's range of accommodation.

10. The child's older cousin, Prentice Rewel, has 5 D hyperopia with a 10 D amplitude of accommodation. What is his near point and range of accommodation when he is not wearing spectacles? What about when he is wearing +5 D spectacles?

Without spectacles: near point = 20 cm, range = infinity to 20 cm; with spectacles: near point = 10 cm, range = infinity to 10 cm.

Without spectacles, he must use 5 D to correct the underlying hyperopia and see at infinity. As such, he only has 5 D left to see at near:

Near point: 1/5 D = 0.20 m = 20 cm; Range of accommodation: infinity to 20 cm (Fig. 9.2).

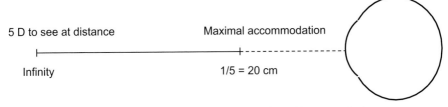

Fig. 9.2 Prentice's range of accommodation without spectacles.

With spectacles, he can still see at infinity, but can now use the full 10 D of accommodative amplitude to see at near:

Near point: 1/10 D = 0.10 m = 10 cm; Range of accommodation: infinity to 10 cm (Fig. 9.3).

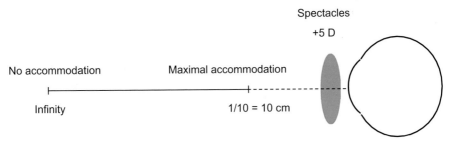

Fig. 9.3 Prentice's range of accommodation with spectacles.

11. **The child's mother, Lady Frenella Prism, has 15 D myopia with a 10 D amplitude of accommodation. What is her range of accommodation with spectacles? What about without spectacles?**

With spectacles: infinity to 10 cm; without spectacles: 6.7 cm to 4.0 cm.

With spectacles, Frenella is in focus at infinity when accommodation is relaxed. When she maximally accommodates, she can use all 10 D to see at near, so she is in focus at 1/10 D = 0.1 m = 10 cm in front of the eye. As such, her range of accommodation is infinity to 10 cm.

Without spectacles, things are different in myopia versus hyperopia. Those with uncorrected myopia have a far point that is not at infinity. Think of it as a "head start" on accommodation. In Frenella's case, her uncorrected 15 D of myopia is like 15 D of built-in accommodation. Thus her farthest point of clear vision without correction is 1/15 D = 6.7 cm in front of the eye. When she does accommodate, the 10 D that she can generate adds to the 15 D that is already built in, and her near point is 1/25 D = 0.040 m = 4 cm. As such, her range of accommodation is 6.7 cm to 4.0 cm (Fig. 9.4).

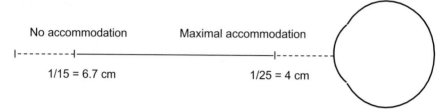

Fig. 9.4 Lady Frenella's range of accommodation without spectacles (with uncorrected myopia → far point is not at infinity).

12. **The child's great-grandfather, Conrad F. Sturm, has a range of accommodation of 20 cm to 12.5 cm without spectacles. What is his amplitude of accommodation? What is his distance refraction? What is his range of accommodation with spectacles?**

   Accommodative amplitude: 3 D; distance refraction: −5 D; range of accommodation with spectacles: infinity to 33 cm.

   To calculate the amplitude of accommodation, calculate the diopters needed to see at the two distances:

   > Far point: 20 cm → 1/0.20 = 5 D
   > Near point: 12.5 cm → 1/0.125 = 8 D
   > Accommodative amplitude: 8 D − 5 D = 3 D

   With accommodation completely relaxed, he is in focus at 20 cm (the far point). The reciprocal of this distance is his refraction (1/0.2 m) = 5 D. Ignoring vertex distance, his distance correction is therefore −5 D. With −5 D glasses on, he is functionally emmetropic, so his far point is infinity. With full accommodation of 3 D, he can see to 1/3 D = 0.33 m = 33 cm. His range of accommodation with spectacles is infinity to 33 cm.

13. **The child's uncle, Gil Strand, can see 20/20 at distance and clearly at near up to 50 cm. With a +3 D addition, he can see clearly from 1 m to 20 cm.**

   (a) **What is his accommodative amplitude?**

   4 D.

   This is a tough accommodation question (and, as such, a good one for exams!). To calculate accommodative amplitude, you need to calculate the dioptric equivalent at both ends of an accommodative range. Be careful: if a patient can see clearly at infinity, you cannot know if some of the accommodation is being used to correct underlying hyperopia (or overcorrected myopia). Therefore ignore the range with infinity (infinity → 50 cm) and use the known range with +3 D (1 m → 20 cm).

   > Far point = 100 cm = 1 m → 1 D
   > Near point = 20 cm = 0.20 m → 5 D
   > Accommodative amplitude = 5 D − 1 D = 4 D

(b) What is his refractive error?

2 D of hyperopia.

A person with emmetropia with 4 D of accommodative amplitude would be able to see clearly to 1/4 m = 0.25 m = 25 cm. Since he can only see to 50 cm, he must have underlying refractive error. Of his 4 D of accommodative amplitude, he is only able to use 2 D to see to 50 cm, so the other 2 D must be needed to see at infinity. He thus has 2 D of underlying hyperopia.

(c) What single vision reading glasses should you give him to read comfortably at 33 cm?

3 D.

To read comfortably, he can use half of his accommodative amplitude of 4 D → 2 D. Since he has 2 D hyperopia, all 2 D must be used to correct his underlying refractive error, and reading glasses must give him all of the power needed to see at near. The power required is 1/0.33 m = 3 D for reading glasses.

(d) What bifocal add should you give him to read comfortably at 33 cm?

1 D.

To read comfortably, he can use half of his accommodative amplitude of 4 D; that is, 2 D. With his glasses on, no accommodation is needed to see at distance, so he can use the entire 2 D to read. Since he needs a total of 3 D to see at 33 cm, he will need an additional 1 D add in his bifocal.

EXAM PEARL

For an exam question, you can assume that a person can use *half* of their accommodative amplitude comfortably (unless explicitly stated otherwise). Use this assumption for questions about prescribing reading glasses or bifocals. Also, be careful not to assume that a patient has emmetropia or is fully corrected. A patient who can see clearly at infinity may still have undercorrected hyperopia (or overcorrected myopia). Patients with undercorrected hyperopia must use up some of their accommodative amplitude to see at distance, and as a result, they cannot use their full accommodative amplitude to see at near.

14. **Stu Deus, a 26-year-old student, is having trouble seeing at near. His structural eye exam is normal, but his accommodative amplitude is only 1 D. What are some possible reasons?**

There are many potential causes of inadequate accommodation:
- *Lens changes:* normal presbyopia
- Impaired accommodation
  - Congenital, idiopathic accommodative insufficiency
  - Oral medication
    - Parasympatholytics, phenothiazines, tranquilizers, and chloroquines
  - Systemic factors
    - Systemic illnesses (e.g., hypothyroidism, severe anemia, myasthenia gravis, and diabetes)

- Down syndrome
- Prior encephalitis or meningitis
- Trauma
  - Head trauma/concussion
  - Eye trauma
- Local factors
  - Tonic pupil
  - Cycloplegic use

15. **Lacy Aigh, a 21-year-old college junior, presents to your clinic 1 week before her final exams with a new-onset intermittent esotropia associated with poor distance vision. What is the most likely diagnosis and what would you do to help confirm it? How about treatment?**

It is likely a *spasm of accommodation*. Look for small pupils and a myopic shift when she is esotropic to confirm the diagnosis. Perform a complete examination to rule out other causes. Explain the problem to the patient and try to alleviate her fears. Ask her to look away from her near work frequently to relax accommodation and/or offer reading glasses/bifocals. A trial of cycloplegia (such as 1% atropine) can also be tried to break the accommodative spasm. Some patients with refractory accommodative spasm require psychiatric care for treatment.

16. **Studs McStudley, a 45-year-old man with −10 D of myopia, decides he would like to try contact lenses after a lifetime of wearing glasses. He tries trial contact lenses and arranges for a Tinder date. However, he says that not only did he have trouble reading the small print in the Tinder user agreement on his phone, but he also found that he did not see the date's features clearly and was rather surprised at the date's actual appearance. Why might he be having trouble?**

When a person with myopia switches from glasses to contact lenses (or has refractive surgery), there are two things that can make near work more challenging:

(1) *Increased accommodative demand*: When a person with myopia wears glasses, the distance from a near object to the spectacle plane is shorter than the distance from the near object to the cornea or contact lens. Therefore the light is less divergent at the point where it is refracted. The result is that changing from myopic glasses to myopic contact lenses increases the accommodative demand. This effect can be proven with example calculations, but it is usually enough to know the concept. Conversely, a person with hyperopia has greater accommodative demand through glasses compared with contact lenses.

(2) *Increased convergence demand*: When a patient with myopia reads through glasses, the eyes converge such that the line of sight is nasal to the optical center of the glasses. This provides a small amount of base-in prism (see Prentice's rule in Chapter 16, Prisms and Diplopia), which aids convergence. When the glasses are removed, the convergence aid is lost, and the demand for convergence is greater. The opposite is true in hyperopia. This effect is less important than the accommodative effect, but easier to figure out in case you forget the answer to part 1 of this question.

CHAPTER 10

Cylinders, Crosses (Axis and Power), and Spherocylindrical Notation

1. **On the first day of her pediatric ophthalmology rotation, resident Halpme Pulease picks up a +3 D cylinder trial lens and holds it with the axis at 90 degrees. How could she describe the cylinder (using axis and power)? Draw the axis cross and power cross for this cylinder.**

    See Fig. 10.1. The cylinder appears to be flat along its vertical meridian. This is the axis. The curvature is along the horizontal meridian. This is the power.

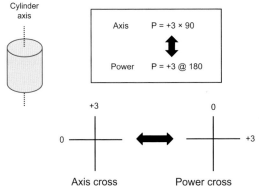

Fig. 10.1 Cylinder notation in terms of axis and power. Axis is indicated by an "x"/Power is indicated by an "@" sign. Axis and Power are always perpendicular.

EXAM PEARL

The orientation of cylinders can be confusing. By convention, a cylinder is defined by its *axis* (likely because this is how we physically see a cylinder). The power is always perpendicular to (90 degrees away from) the axis. The power is what is acting on the light, but the axis is what we use to describe the cylinder. To add to the confusion, the power acts on parallel light to create a focal line that is parallel to the axis (Fig. 10.2). It is important to keep this in mind for any question involving cylinders. Read carefully to look for axis versus power in the question (and in the answer options for multiple-choice questions).

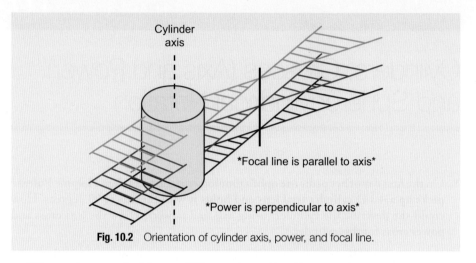

Fig. 10.2 Orientation of cylinder axis, power, and focal line.

2. What is the conoid of Sturm? What is the circle of least confusion?

When light passes through a spherocylindrical (astigmatic) lens, it is focused not to a point, but into two successive focal lines. Each focal line is formed by the power of the lens acting in the meridian that is at a right angle to the focal line (i.e., the focal lines are *perpendicular to the power* and *parallel to the axes* of the lens). The envelope formed by these rays of light changes from an elliptical shape in one orientation to an elliptical shape 90 degrees away; this envelope is referred to as the *conoid of Sturm* (Fig. 10.3).

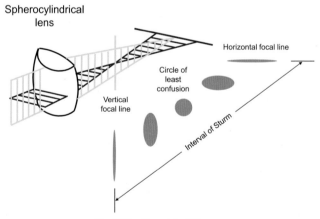

Fig. 10.3 Conoid of Sturm.

The average dioptric power of the lens, called the *spherical equivalent* of the lens, is associated with a plane halfway between the two focal lines (in diopters, *not* distance). Letters are theoretically easiest to recognize at this point, as the blur is equal in all meridians. For this reason, this location is referred to as the *circle of least confusion*; it is a circle because its perimeter is defined by the round pupil aperture.

The conoid of Sturm is outlined by the lens aperture and includes two focal lines at each end and the circle of least confusion in between (Fig. 10.3).

3. **Convert the glasses prescription +1.00 +2.00 × 80 to minus cylinder notation.**

Minus cylinder notation: +3.00 −2.00 × 170

Every spherocylindrical lens has two equivalent notations: a plus cylinder notation and a minus cylinder notation. To convert from plus to minus cylinder (or vice versa), follow these three steps:
1. New sphere = old sphere + old cylinder
2. New cylinder = same as old cylinder but opposite sign
3. New axis = change old axis by 90 degrees

For this lens:
1. New sphere = +1.00 +2.00 → +3.00
2. New cylinder = +2.00 → −2.00
3. New axis = 80 degrees + 90 degrees → 170 degrees
So, +1.00 +2.00 × 80 ↔ +3.00 −2.00 × 170

4. **What is the spherical equivalent of −1.00 +2.00 × 45? What type of cylinder is this?**

Spherical equivalent: Plano; Jackson cross cylinder.

The formula for spherical equivalent is:

> spherical equivalent (SE) (in diopters) = sphere + (1/2) cylinder

So, spherical equivalent (SE) = −1.00 + (1/2)2.00 = −1.00 + 1.00 = 0 → plano

This happens to describe a ±1 D Jackson cross cylinder. A Jackson cross cylinder is a special type of cylinder with spherical equivalent = plano (by definition), which is used to help refine cylinder axis and power during subjective refraction. Note that the Jackson cross cylinder is defined by the sphere power in spherocylindrical notation, which is the same as the power on either meridian of the power cross, so this is a ±1 D Jackson cross cylinder, *not* a ±2 D Jackson cross cylinder.

5. **Write a prescription for a ±0.50 D Jackson cross cylinder (plus and minus cylinder notation). Why are Jackson cross cylinders available with a variety of powers?**

$$+0.50 - 1.00 \times 90 \, (\text{minus cylinder notation})$$
$$-0.50 + 1.00 \times 180 \, (\text{plus cylinder notation})$$

Note that the axis is specified at random (it depends on how you are holding the cylinder). As long as the axis of the minus cylinder notation is 90 degrees away from that of the plus cylinder notation, you have the correct answer.

Patients with poor visual acuity need to be shown a bigger difference for comparison when subjectively refining cylinder axis and power. A ±0.25 D Jackson cross cylinder is built into most phoropters and is suitable for most people, optimizing refinement of the refraction as it approaches 20/25. Jackson cross cylinder options include ±0.12 D (20/15 to 20/20), ±0.25 D (20/25 to 20/30), ±0.50 D (20/40 to 20/60), and ±1.00 D (20/70 to 20/200).

6. **During a subjective refraction, you increase the cylinder by +0.50 D. How much should you change the sphere and in which direction? Why?**

   Change the sphere by –0.25 D. This keeps the spherical equivalent the same.

   For any change in cylinder, you must change the sphere by half as much and in the opposite direction to keep the spherical equivalent the same. This keeps the circle of least confusion on the retina during refraction. So, if you add +0.50 D of cylinder, you should change the sphere by –0.25 D. Similarly, if you are refracting in minus cylinder and you add –0.50 cylinder, you should change the sphere by +0.25 D.

7. **What is the spherocylindrical notation, both plus and minus, for the combination of the following two cylindrical lenses:**

   Lens #1: + 3.00 × 170

   Lens #2: −5.25 × 80

   +3.00 −8.25 × 80   or   −5.25 +8.25 × 170

   There are a number of different approaches to this type of a problem. All work fine. One way may seem more reasonable to you than another depending on your problem-solving style. Three approaches are presented next.

   Method 1: Use axis crosses
   This method can be used to determine minus cylinder (Fig. 10.4) or plus cylinder (Fig. 10.5) spherocylindrical notation (can also be done using power crosses).

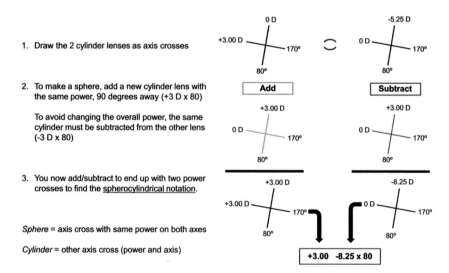

Fig. 10.4 Axis cross method for combining cylinders (+3.00 × 170 and –5.25 × 80) into spherocylindrical notation (minus cylinder option).

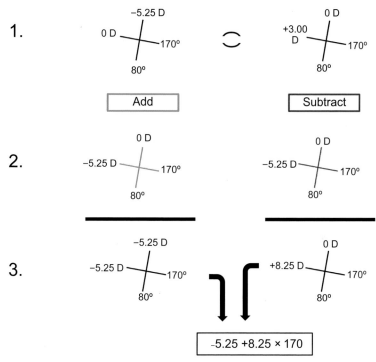

Fig. 10.5 Axis cross method for combining cylinders (+3.00 × 170 and −5.25 × 80) into spherocylindrical notation (plus cylinder option).

Method 2: Add/subtract lens powers

1. Take one of the cylinders and add a new cylinder of equal power with axis 90 degrees away. This gives you the sphere (with power equal to the power of the first cylinder).
2. The cylinder that was added in Step 1 must now be subtracted to keep the lens the same. Take the other original cylinder and subtract the cylinder you added in Step 1. This gives you the power and axis of the cylinder:

$$+3.00 \times 170 \text{ combined with } -5.25 \times 80$$

1. Take 1 cylinder: $+3.00 \times 170$

   Add new cylinder to get sphere: $\underline{+3.00 \times 80}$

                                                              $+3$ sphere

2. Take other cylinder: -5.25×80

   Subtract cylinder that was added: $\underline{-3.00 \times 80}$

                                                              -8.25×80 cylinder

   Spherocylindrical lens: $+3.00 -8.25 \times 80$

Method 3: Quick "in your head" method

Here is another three-step method that involves more memorization but requires less understanding.

1. Select one lens and declare that it will be the spherical part of the spherocylindrical lens.
2. Now ask, how many diopters must be added or subtracted to obtain the power in the other meridian?
3. Finally, which axis specifies the meridian requiring this additional power?

In the previous question:

1. Make lens #1 the sphere (sphere = +3.00 D)
2. Calculate the diopters required to get to the other meridian (+3.00 → −5.25 = −8.25 D).
3. Finally, at which axis (×80)

This gives you the spherocylindrical notation: +3.00 −8.25 × 80. If you started with −5.25 D = sphere, you would get the plus cylinder form: −5.25 +8.25 × 170.

All methods can be used to convert two cylinders into a spherocylindrical lens. Choose whichever method makes the most sense to you and then apply it consistently. It is important to practice (see Question 8). To check your work, convert your spherocylindrical lens back into a power cross (or axis cross) and ensure that it is the same as the original combination of two cylindrical lenses.

8. **Convert the axis and power crosses in Fig. 10.6 to spherocylindrical notation (i.e., spectacle correction). Give both plus and minus cylinder notations.**

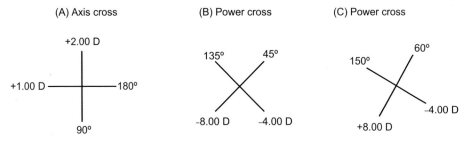

Fig. 10.6   Axis and power crosses.

(a) Plus cylinder form: +1.00 +1.00 × 90
    Minus cylinder form: +2.00 −1.00 × 180
(b) Plus cylinder form: −8.00 +4.00 × 45
    Minus cylinder form: −4.00 −4.00 × 135
(c) Plus cylinder form: −4.00 +12.00 × 150
    Minus cylinder form: +8.00 −12.00 × 60

9. Convert the spherocylindrical lens +5.00 –1.00 × 180 into a power cross and axis cross.

See Fig. 10.7. Converting spherocylindrical notation to power and axis crosses is a key skill. There are also several methods to do this. It does not matter which you use, as long as you can do it quickly and accurately. Do not be discouraged by the multiple methods, just focus on one that speaks to you and stick with it.

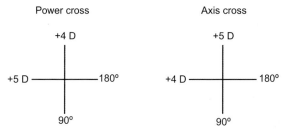

Fig. 10.7   Power cross and axis cross of the lens +5.00 –1.00 × 180.

Method 1: Split the sphere and add the cylinders (Fig. 10.8)

1. *Divide the sphere* of the lens into a power cross of two cylinders (same power as sphere with one axis the same as the cylinder axis and the other axis 90 degrees away).
2. *Convert the cylinder* of the lens into a power cross.
3. *Adding the power crosses together* gives you the power cross of the glasses.
4. The power cross can be converted into the axis cross by flipping the powers (axes stay the same).

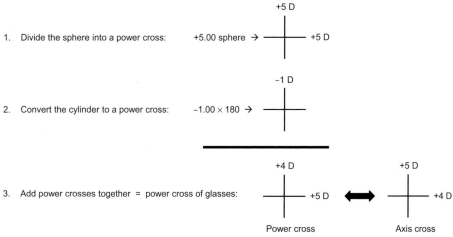

Fig. 10.8   Method 1 for converting spherocylindrical notation (+5.00 –1.00 × 180) to a power cross (and axis cross).

Method 2: Method of spheres (Fig. 10.9)

1. Calculate the plus cylinder and minus cylinder forms of the spherocylindrical lens.
2. Take the power of sphere and cylinder axis of the plus cylinder form → place on power cross.
3. Do the same for the minus cylinder form (power and axis) → place on power cross.

Plus cylinder form: +4.00 +1.00 × 90° → +4.00 @ 90

Minus cylinder form: +5.00 –1.00 × 180° → +5.00 @ 180

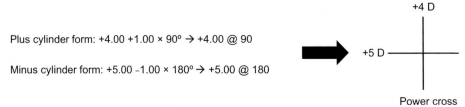

Fig. 10.9   Method 2 for converting spherocylindrical notation (+5.00 –1.00 × 180) to a power cross.

Method 3: Do it in your head (Fig. 10.10)

Quicker but requires more mental gymnastics. To calculate the power cross:

1. One axis = the power of the sphere with the same axis as the spherocylindrical notation.
2. Other axis = the power equal to the sphere + cylinder, with axis 90 degrees away from original axis.

1. One axis = sphere power and original axis → +5.00 @ 180

2. Other axis = add sphere + cylinder, axis 90 away → +4.00 @ 90

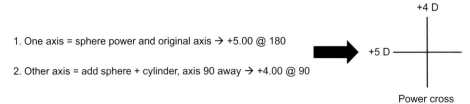

Fig. 10.10   Method 3 for converting spherocylindrical notation (+5.00 –1.00 × 180) to a power cross.

EXAM PEARL

Remember that for a cylinder, the axis provides power in a meridian 90 degrees away (axis and power are perpendicular). Some people prefer to work strictly with power crosses; just be careful to add or subtract 90 degrees when writing the spectacle prescription (glasses are always written with axis by convention). Others find that they are less likely to confuse meridians by converting the power cross to an axis cross before making any other calculations. The axis cross is easiest to use when doing retinoscopy with free spherical lenses. Whatever you use, always *label carefully*!

---

10. **Convert the following prescriptions to plus or minus cylinder notation. Compute the spherical equivalent and draw the power cross and axis cross.**

    (a) +3.00 −2.00 × 80

(b) +1.00 −4.00 × 80

(c) −5.00 +9.00 × 90

(a) +3.00 −2.00 × 80 → +1.00 +2.00 × 170 (plus cylinder notation); spherical equivalent +2.00 D. Power and axis cross (answer Fig. 10.11).

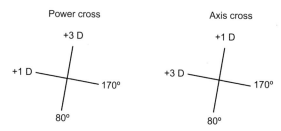

Fig. 10.11   Power cross and axis cross for Question 10(a).

(b) +1.00 −4.00 × 80 → −3.00 +4.00 × 170 (plus cylinder notation); spherical equivalent −1.00 D. Power and axis cross (answer Fig. 10.12).

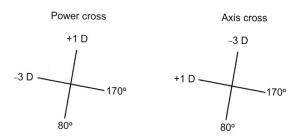

Fig. 10.12   Power cross and axis cross for Question 10(b).

(c) −5.00 +9.00 × 90 → +4.00 −9.00 × 180 (minus cylinder notation); spherical equivalent −0.50 D. Power and axis cross (answer Fig. 10.13).

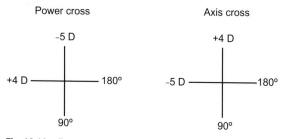

Fig. 10.13   Power cross and axis cross for Question 10(c).

11. **For each of the following lenses in Fig. 10.14, calculate the spherical equivalent. How far are the two focal lines and the circle of least confusion from the lens, assuming a point object arising at infinity?**

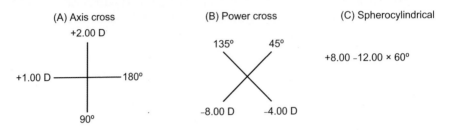

(A) Axis cross

(B) Power cross

(C) Spherocylindrical

+8.00 –12.00 × 60°

Fig. 10.14 Example lenses.

Lens (A): Circle of least confusion: +0.67 m; spherical equivalent: +1.50 D; focal line at 180 degrees: +1 m; focal line at 90 degrees: +0.50 m.

Lens (B): Circle of least confusion: −0.167 m; spherical equivalent: −6.00 D; focal line at 135 degrees: −0.125 m; focal line at 45 degrees: −0.25 m.

Lens (C): Circle of least confusion: +0.50 m; spherical equivalent: +2.00 D; focal line at 150 degrees: +0.125 m; focal line at 60 degrees: −0.25 m.

Remember, spherical equivalent = (sphere) + (1/2 × cylinder)

To calculate the location of the circle of least confusion, take the reciprocal of the spherical equivalent (the circle of least confusion is *not* geometrically halfway in between the focal lines). To calculate the location of focal lines, take the reciprocal of the cylinder powers (the focal lines are parallel to the axis/perpendicular to the power).

(a) Spherical equivalent = (+1.00) + (1/2) × (+1.00) = +1.50. The circle of least confusion is at the focal plane of the spherical equivalent (1/+1.50) = +0.67 m. The plus sign indicates that it is to the right of the lens. The focal line in the 180-degree meridian is formed by the power acting 90 degrees away, in the 90-degree meridian. Since the power in the 90-degree meridian is +1.00 D, the focal line in the 180-degree meridian will be formed 1 m to the right of the lens. Similarly, the focal line in the 90-degree meridian is (1/2) = 0.5 m away.

(b) The negative distances mean that the focal lines and circle of least confusion are all to the left of the lens.

(c) The focal line at 150 degrees is 0.125 m to the right of the lens and the focal line at 60 degrees is 0.25 m to the left of the lens.

12. **A spherocylindrical lens converts light from a point object at infinity to a horizontal line at +0.33 m and a vertical line at +0.5 m. Draw the power cross for the lens. With light traveling from left to right through the lens, where is the circle**

of least confusion for the conoid of Sturm thus formed? What is the spherocylindrical notation for this lens (plus and minus cylinder notation)?

See Fig. 10.15.

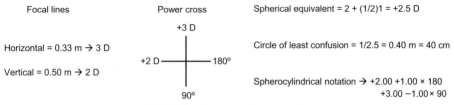

Focal lines

Horizontal = 0.33 m → 3 D

Vertical = 0.50 m → 2 D

Power cross

+3 D

+2 D —————— 180°

90°

Spherical equivalent = 2 + (1/2)1 = +2.5 D

Circle of least confusion = 1/2.5 = 0.40 m = 40 cm

Spherocylindrical notation → +2.00 +1.00 × 180
+3.00 −1.00 × 90

Fig. 10.15 Answer to Question 12.

CHAPTER 11

Astigmatism

1. **In Fig. 11.1, the two focal lines for eyes with astigmatic refractive error are indicated by short lines. What types of ametropia are represented in the figure?**

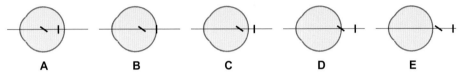

A   **B**   **C**   **D**   **E**

Fig. 11.1 Types of ametropia.

The types of ametropia are:
(A) Compound myopic astigmatism
(B) Simple myopic astigmatism
(C) Mixed astigmatism
(D) Simple hyperopic astigmatism
(E) Compound hyperopic astigmatism

2. **A patient wears glasses with power +1.00 +2.00 × 90. Is this "with-the-rule" astigmatism or "against-the-rule" astigmatism and why? What do you call astigmatism that is neither with nor against the rule?**

This is with-the-rule astigmatism; oblique astigmatism is not "with-the-rule" or "against-the-rule".

With-the-rule astigmatism means that the vertical corneal meridian is steepest. With-the-rule astigmatism is corrected with plus cylinder at 90 degrees (or minus cylinder at 180 degrees). The axis does not have to be exactly 90 degrees or 180 degrees; within 20 degrees on either side qualifies (i.e., correcting plus cylinder axis 70 degrees to 110 degrees). Against-the-rule astigmatism means that the horizontal corneal meridian is steepest, such that the correcting plus cylinder is at 180 degrees (or minus cylinder at 90 degrees), again within the range of ±20 degrees (correcting plus cylinder axis 160 degrees to 20 degrees). Outside of those limits, the ametropia is referred to as *oblique astigmatism*.

3. **What type of astigmatism do children usually have? What about older adults?**

Children: with-the-rule; Older adults: against-the-rule.

Children tend to have with-the-rule astigmatism. This may be due to the elasticity of the eyelids in children or the pliability of the cornea. The tight lids press down on the upper and lower cornea and steepen its vertical meridian. Older adults have flabby, stretched-out eyelids, and thus they tend to have against-the-rule astigmatism. . . at least until a cataract or refractive surgery mishap converts the astigmatism back to with-the-rule (and makes them feel young again!).

4. **For the following glasses prescription, what type of astigmatism is present: Compound or simple hyperopic or myopic, or mixed? With-the-rule, against-the-rule, or oblique?**

   (a) $+3.00 - 2.00 \times 80$

   (b) $+1.00 - 4.00 \times 175$

   (c) $-5.00 + 9.00 \times 65$

   (a) Compound hyperopic astigmatism, against-the-rule
   (b) Mixed astigmatism, with-the-rule
   (c) Mixed astigmatism, oblique

   If we write (a) in plus cylinder notation, the result is $+1.00 +2.00 \times 170$. Since the spere is positive in both notations, it is compound hyperopic astigmatism. The axis of minus cylinder is close to 90 degrees, so it is against-the-rule. For (b), the prescription in plus cylinder notation is $-3.00 +4.00 \times 85$; since the sphere number is positive in one notation and negative in the other, it is mixed astigmatism. We will leave it to you to figure out the rest of the answers.

EXAM PEARL

To determine the type of astigmatism a patient has from their glasses, write out the plus and minus cylinder forms of the lenses. You can then use the sign of the power of the spheres to assess the type of astigmatism (Table 11.1).

TABLE 11.1 ▪ Method Using Sign of Spheres to Assess Type of Astigmatism

Spherical Powers in Plus and Minus Cylinder Forms	Type of Astigmatism
Both positive	Compound hyperopic
Both negative	Compound myopic
Plano and positive	Simple hyperopic
Plano and negative	Simple myopic
One positive, one negative	Mixed

5. **Orson Nist is something of a firebug. He wears glasses of $+3.00 +2.00 \times 90$ in both eyes.**

   (a) **Orson decides it is time to start a fire, but he forgot to bring his matches. Instead, he removes his glasses and angles them toward the sun in an effort** to focus the light and initiate a flame. **What he sees instead are focal lines and a circle of least confusion, neither of which seem to be focused well enough to cause any damage. Where are the focal lines and the circle of least confusion with respect to the lenses in this case?**

Vertical focal line: 20 cm behind the lens; horizontal focal line: 33 cm behind the lens; circle of least confusion: 25 cm behind the lens (Fig. 11.2).

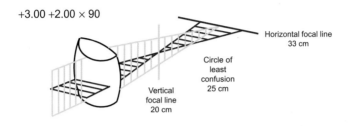

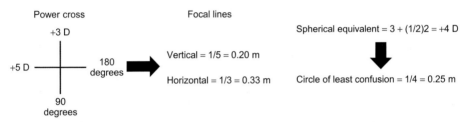

Fig. 11.2   Location of focal lines and circle of least confusion for lens +3.00 +2.00 × 90.

This is a good example of how the circle of least confusion is not geometrically halfway between the two focal lines (that would be at 26.5 cm behind the lens). Instead, it is dioptrically halfway between the focal lines, which is why you need to calculate the spherical equivalent and take the reciprocal.

(b) With his glasses still in his hand, Orson looks directly at the sun to be sure that the sun itself is not the reason that he cannot start a fire with his glasses. With his accommodation completely relaxed, where are the focal lines and circle of least confusion in relation to the retina while he is gazing at the sun?

Both focal lines and the circle of least confusion are just behind the retina (a few millimeters). The horizontal line is closest to the retina and the vertical focal line is further behind, with the circle of least confusion in-between.

This demonstrates the difference between where focal lines lie for a corrective lens versus the eye itself. For a corrective lens, the focal lines are simply the reciprocal of the values on the power cross. For the eye itself, the focal lines are based on the error created by deviations in the power of the model eye, about 60 D. In general, to estimate the distance of the focal point from the retina, you can use the rule-of-thumb that it is about 1 mm for every 2 to 3 D of refractive error. To be more exact, we can modify Orson's schematic eye to include an error lens for his hyperopia (Fig. 11.3).

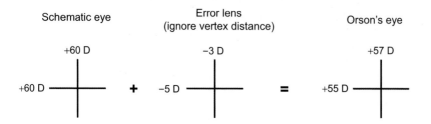

Schematic eye emmetropic retina: 1/60 = 0.1666 m = 16.7 mm behind the nodal point

Horizontal focal line: 1/57 = 17.5 mm behind the nodal point, or 0.9 mm behind the retina

Vertical focal line: 1/55 = 18.2 mm behind the nodal point, or 1.5 mm behind the retina

Circle of least confusion: 1/56 = 17.9 mm behind the nodal point, or 1.2 mm behind the retina

Fig. 11.3 Estimated location of focal lines in relation to the retina in an eye with compound hyperopia (using the reduced schematic eye and error lens).

6. **You are performing retinoscopy on a child at a distance of 2/3 m. When you orient the streak in the horizontal meridian and sweep vertically, you neutralize the reflex with a +3.00 D lens. When you orient the streak in the vertical meridian and sweep horizontally, you neutralize the reflex with a +4.00 D lens. What glasses prescription would you prescribe to fully correct this refractive error? What would the prescription be if your working distance was 1/2 m?**

+1.50 +1.00 × 90 at 2/3 m
+1.00 +1.00 × 90 at 1/2 m

The retinoscopy results are easiest to summarize with an axis cross. First, you sweep the horizontal streak up/down. This is checking the power in the vertical meridian (horizontal axis). Next, you sweep the vertical streak left/right. This is checking the power in the horizontal meridian (vertical axis) (Fig. 11.4). This translates to a spherocylindrical correction of +3.00 +1.00 × 90 (remember, you drew an axis cross, so you do not change the cylinder axis when converting from the cross to a glasses prescription). Don't forget to subtract your working distance (Fig. 11.5). If it is 2/3 m (0.67 m), you need to subtract 1/0.67 = 1.50 D, so the refraction is +1.50 +1.00 × 90. If it is 1/2 m (0.50 m), you need to subtract 1/0.5 = 2.00 D, so the refraction is +1.00 +1.00 × 90.

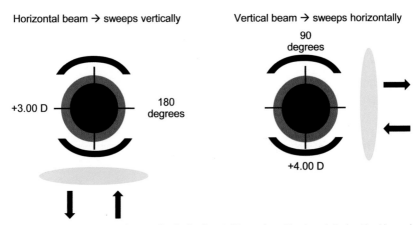

Fig. 11.4 Retinoscopy, sweeping vertically (horizontal beam) and horizontally (vertical beam), the axis of the correcting cylinder is parallel to the beam.

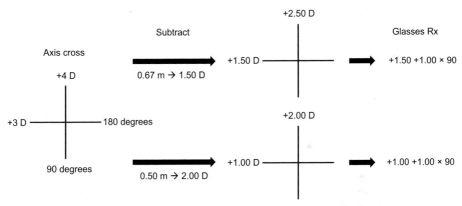

Fig. 11.5 Adjustment for working distance to calculate final refraction.

EXAM PEARL

For any question about cycloplegic retinoscopy, there are two variables to watch out for:

1. *Orientation of beam versus direction of sweep.* The orientation is always perpendicular to the direction of sweep. The question will usually specify (e.g., "with the beam oriented horizontally" or "sweeping vertically"). This is important because the power you place on the axis cross is parallel to the beam orientation and perpendicular to the direction of sweep.

2. *Working distance.* You must adjust for your working distance to get the final refraction by subtracting 1/working distance (in m). If not specified, you can assume a working distance of 0.67 m (take off 1.50 D from each axis to get the final refraction).

7. **After a penetrating keratoplasty, the following keratometry readings are obtained:**
   40 D @ 30°
   43 D @ 120°

(a) **What power and axis of cylindrical correction is required to correct the postoperative astigmatism, assuming all astigmatism is corneal?**

−3.00 × 30   or   +3.00 × 120

There is a 3 D difference between meridians. Ignoring vertex distance, this is corrected with a 3 D cylindrical spectacle lens. The 120-degree meridian is the steepest; thus it has the most plus power. It would be neutralized by −3.00 D of power in that meridian. But astigmatic refractive power exerted in the 120-degree meridian has its axis 90 degrees away (at 30 degrees). Thus, the glasses should have −3.00 × 30 (or +3.00 × 120).

(b) **What is the glasses prescription if you know that the spherical equivalent of the refraction is +1.00 D (ignore vertex distance)?**

+2.50 −3.00 × 30   or   −0.50 +3.00 × 120

A plano spherical equivalent of the required cylindrical correction is +1.50 −3.00 × 30, or −1.50 +3.00 × 120. For a spherical equivalent of +1.00, add +1.00 to the sphere. So the prescription would be +2.50 −3.00 × 30 (or −0.50 +3.00 × 120).

(c) **How does a tight suture change the corneal curvature and why?**

A tight suture steepens the K in the meridian of the suture.

A tight suture flattens the area immediately under the suture. However, the circumference of the globe is constant. Therefore flattening in one area must be balanced by steepening elsewhere in the globe. This compensatory steepening takes place in the center of the cornea overlying the pupil (Fig. 11.6). Try this demonstration: Hold an index card horizontally, giving it a gentle convex curvature. Now without moving the edges of the card, flatten a small section near one edge (this is the tight suture). Note how the rest of the card becomes steeper.

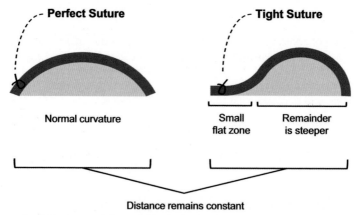

Fig. 11.6   How a tight peripheral suture steepens the central cornea.

(d) Assuming a single, tight, radially placed suture is present, in what meridian would you be most likely to find it? What can you do to improve the corneal astigmatism?

120 degrees → cut the suture at 11:00.

In this example, the tight suture would be at the steepest meridian, which is at 120 degrees (11:00). This suture can be cut to improve the astigmatism. A helpful bit of advice might be the penetrating keratoplasty (PKP) surgeon mantra, "cut the high K."

8. **A 35-year-old man returns to your office 1 hour after receiving the spectacles you prescribed for him. He had never worn glasses before. He says the whole world is like a fishbowl, he feels that the floor is coming up at him, doors are falling toward him, he is dizzy, and has a headache. Visual acuity is 20/50 in each eye without correction and 20/20 in each eye with correction.**

(a) What's wrong?

This is likely due to oblique astigmatism in one or both eyes. Correction of oblique astigmatism can cause subtle distortion under monocular viewing conditions but tremendous distortion of depth under binocular conditions. The easiest example to consider is a door frame. If astigmatic correction is with- or against-the-rule, the door frame may look elongated or shortened but the left side will be just as tall as the right side. With correction of oblique astigmatism, the right eye may see the door frame tilted slightly to the right, which may or may not be noticeable. However, if the left eye sees the door frame tilted slightly to the left, then the binocular visual system (which is sensitive to extremely small disparities between the two eyes) kicks in. The brain will think that the top of the door is closer to the patient than the bottom. He will feel that it is falling toward him (Fig. 11.7). Another possibility is that there is anisometropia with aniseikonia.

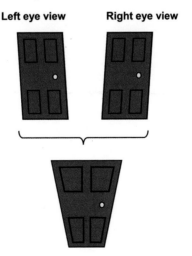

Binocular system interprets door as tilting forward

Fig. 11.7 Depth distortion resulting from binocular oblique astigmatism.

(b) How can this be helped?

There are several options, some which will not affect visual acuity and some which may.

Options that *do not* affect visual acuity:
- Reassure the patient that he will get used to it (the younger the patient and the lower the astigmatism, the more likely this will be true).
- Minimize vertex distance.
- Be sure the lenses are of minus cylinder type (cylinder ground on the back surface of the spectacle lens).
- Consider contact lenses or refractive surgery.

Options that may compromise visual acuity:
- Rotate the cylinder toward the 90-degree or 180-degree meridian.
- Decrease the power of the cylinder.

CHAPTER 12

Aberrations, Distortions, and Irregularities

1. **What is spherical aberration? How does it change refractive error? In what light conditions does spherical aberration have the greatest impact on the refraction of the eye?**

   Rays that strike the periphery of a spherical lens are more strongly bent than rays that strike closer to the center of the lens (i.e., spherical lenses have "positive" spherical aberration). This effectively shortens the focal length of that lens (Fig. 12.1).

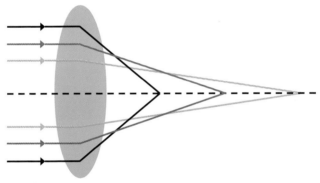

Fig. 12.1 (Positive) spherical aberration: peripheral rays are bent more strongly than central rays.

   With positive spherical aberration, the peripheral rays are refracted more than the central rays, causing the patient to become *more myopic* (or less hyperopic). It also creates distortion. This affects vision most in low light levels when the pupils are more widely dilated.

2. **An ophthalmology resident is performing a cycloplegic retinoscopy on a cooperative 8-year-old child when she notices that the center of the pupil shows a "with" reflex, while the periphery shows "against" movement. What optical phenomenon is responsible? Which reflex should the resident neutralize?**

   Spherical aberration, neutralize the central reflex.

   In a biconvex lens such as the human lens, the peripheral rays are refracted more strongly than the central rays. The peripheral lens thus appears more myopic during retinoscopy than the central lens, especially when the pupil is widely dilated. The resident should neutralize the central reflex, which will be most relevant to the refraction once the dilating drops wear off and the pupil returns to its normal size.

3. **Having just watched a 6-hour optics and refraction YouTube video, you are feeling particularly brave, so you decide to do a full manifest refraction on a young adult with myopia without relying on an autorefractor. At the end of the refraction, you accidentally turn on the duochrome test and decide, "I've gone this far, why not give it a go?"**

   (a) **What aberration is the duochrome test based on?**

   Chromatic aberration.

   The refractive index (n) of transparent materials changes with wavelength. As a result, different wavelengths are bent (refracted) to a different degree based on wavelength: shorter rays (blue, green) are bent more strongly and longer rays (red) are refracted less (Fig. 12.2).

   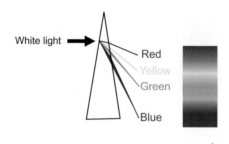

   • Blue is Bent most

   Fig. 12.2   Chromatic aberration.

   (b) **Does the duochrome test work in patients who are color-blind?**

   Yes.

   The test is based on differences in refraction as a function of wavelength, so the patient does not need to perceive true colors for the test to work. Green rays are still bent more strongly than red rays by the lens, so the clarity of the letters will thus be affected even if the patient cannot identify the colors.

   (c) **If the patient sees the letters clearly on the green background but not on the red background, have you overminused or underminused the patient?**

   Overminused.

   Green is refracted more strongly than red, so the red letters are focused more posterior to the lens. If the letters on the green background are clearer, that means the letters on the red background must be behind the retina. When the focal point is behind the retina, the patient is effectively hyperopic; therefore you have overminused the patient and need to cut back on the minus power.

(d) On which side should the letters be clearer at the start of the test? Why?

Red.

The patient should be fogged at the beginning of the test so you can be sure accommodation is relaxed. To do this, you must add plus power until both focal lines are in front of the retina (inside the vitreous), at which point the red (posterior) letters will be closer to the retina and clearer. You then take off plus power until the letters are equally clear, at which point yellow is in focus (optimal for viewing in white light). One way to remember this is that if the patient says, "red is clearer," give more red (minus) power.

4. What is astigmatism of oblique incidence?

Tilting a spherical lens adds both sphere and cylinder of the same sign as the original lens, with the cylinder axis in the axis of the tilt. This is *astigmatism of oblique incidence*. For instance, tilting a −10.00 D lens 10 degrees forward results in −10.10 −0.31 × 180; tilting a +10.00 D lens forward 20 degrees results in +10.41 +1.38 × 180. It is not important to remember the exact amounts of sphere and cylinder induced—just remember that tilting a lens changes both sphere and cylinder power.

5. A senior ophthalmology resident performs retinoscopy on an uncooperative 4-year-old boy and records:

OD: +3.75 +1.00 × 180
OS: +4.50 sphere

The pediatric ophthalmology fellow repeats the retinoscopy and finds +4.50 sphere in each eye. Assuming the fellow's retinoscopy is correct, what is the likely cause of the discrepancy?

Astigmatism of oblique incidence.

During the resident's retinoscopy of the right eye, the child was trying to spit and kick. The resident moved to the patient's right to avoid danger and continued the retinoscopy while the boy was distracted by a toy slightly to his left. This caused astigmatism of oblique incidence, which caused the resident to detect additional plus sphere and plus cylinder induced in the axis of tilt of the boy's eye (90 degrees). As such, the correcting lens had less overall plus power and correcting plus cylinder at axis 180 degrees. The pediatric ophthalmology fellow, who by now is used to being spit on and kicked at, does not feel the need to move out of the way and performed retinoscopy on axis.

6. Why do glasses have a pantoscopic tilt?

To minimize astigmatism of oblique incidence.

Pantoscopic tilt is the forward tilt of the spectacle plane relative to vertical. The curvature and tilt of spectacle lenses are designed to minimize astigmatism of oblique incidence. If spectacle lenses were perpendicular to the horizon, there would be significant astigmatism of oblique incidence in the reading position. If they were optimized for reading position, astigmatism of oblique incidence would be maximal for distance viewing. Pantoscopic tilt is the slight (7-degree) forward tilt of a spectacle lens that is a compromise between the optimal position of the lenses for distance and near work.

7. Why do patients with myopia sometimes tilt their glasses?

To gain minus power.

People with undercorrected myopia often tilt their glasses to gain more minus sphere. People with undercorrected hyperopia could do the same, but they usually slide their glasses down their noses to gain more effective plus power instead. With myopic lenses, additional effective minus power could be achieved by pushing the glasses closer to the eyes, but this is harder to sustain than tilting the lenses.

8. What is coma?

Coma is the off-axis effect of spherical aberration.

Coma causes light rays to be distributed in a pattern like that of a comet. Coma generally increases as an object moves away from the optical axis.

9. A 22-year-old man has been reluctant to pursue strabismus surgery but is complaining that his prism glasses create rainbows when driving at night. While all prism glasses produce rainbows, you suspect a problem with the Abbe value of his lenses. What is the Abbe value and which is better, a high or a low Abbe value?

The Abbe value indicates the degree of chromatic aberration, higher is better (less chromatic aberration).

The Abbe value (or Abbe number) was named after Ernst Abbe, a German physicist. It indicates the degree of chromatic aberration caused by a lens. Lenses with higher Abbe values have less chromatic aberration. (Think of the Abbe value as a board exam score: higher is better.) In this case, you contact the optician and discover that the patient was fitted with polycarbonate lenses, which have an Abbe value of 30. The optician updates the prism glasses with mid-index plastic lenses, which have a similar refractive index and an Abbe value of 47, and the patient reports considerable improvement in the rainbows.

CHAPTER 13

Contact Lenses

1. Describe how you would evaluate a patient who wishes to wear contact lenses.

The steps in this exercise are as follows:
1. Obtain an accurate refraction.
2. If considering a rigid lens, convert to minus cylinder form and drop the minus cylinder (use spherical power only; the tears between the cornea and the contact lens form a cylindrical "lens" that will correct corneal astigmatism).
3. Calculate correction for zero vertex distance.
4. Evaluate the anterior segment with a slit lamp exam:
   ■ Look for corneal edema, vascularization, and staining; note contour.
   ■ Note tear film and tear film breakup time (normally >10 seconds); consider Schirmer testing.
   ■ Look for lid abnormalities, flip the eyelid to check for papillae, and note palpebral fissures.
   ■ Check for an eccentric pupil.
5. Perform keratometry; compare results with spectacle refraction to detect lenticular astigmatism.
6. Discuss available contact lens options with the patient.
7. Fit lenses (see later discussion).

2. How do you evaluate the fit of a rigid versus soft contact lens?

Note: There is no longer a simple dichotomy of rigid versus soft contact lenses. A variety of lenses with specific fitting protocols are currently available. Still, understanding the basics of a rigid versus soft contact lens fit will allow you to make informed recommendations regardless of the available technology.

Rigid lens: Place a drop of fluorescein in the eye to visualize the tears that cushion the contact lens as it sits on the surface of the eye. You should see a localized pool of tears under the center of the lens.

Soft lens: Fluorescein will stain soft contact lenses, and these lenses do not ride atop a tear cushion. Instead, you evaluate the fit of soft lenses by how well they move after a blink. Steep lenses do not move with a blink; flat lenses move too much.

3. A contact lens is labeled 8.9/13.5/+12.50. What do the numbers mean?

Base curve is 8.9 mm (this is the radius of curvature of the lens, the base curve can also be described in terms of power, measured in diopters, though it is more than a simple reciprocal); *diameter* is 13.5 mm; *power* is +12.50 diopters (D).

4. **How many diopters of power correspond to a corneal radius of curvature of 8.9 mm?**

Using the *standard keratometric formula* (derived in Chapter 17, Instruments):

$$P_{cornea} = \frac{0.3375\,m}{r(m)} = \frac{337.5\,mm}{r(mm)} = \frac{337.5\,mm}{8.9\,mm} = 37.9\,D$$

Note that this approximates the overall refractive power of the cornea, based on a standardized conversion factor developed in the 1800s. Keratometry measures the radius of curvature of the anterior corneal surface. The reason the keratometric index of refraction (n = 1.3375) is different than the refractive index of the cornea (n = 1.376) is that it takes into account the minus power of the posterior surface of the cornea. This standardized factor is used so that a 7.5-mm radius of curvature corresponds to exactly 45 D.

5. **Mr. A. Luddite has K readings of 44.50/45.50 and asks to be fitted with a rigid gas permeable contact lens. Having prescribed nothing but soft contact lenses for as long as you remember, you are a bit taken aback, but the patient insists on rigid lenses. You vaguely remember that you are supposed to fit a rigid lens steeper than the lower K.**

(a) **What does it mean to fit the lens "steeper than the lower K"?**

Fitting a lens "steeper than the lower K" means that you choose a lens with a base curve that is greater (often 0.5 D) than the lower K-reading.

(b) **What curvature of lens would you pick to fit a lens 0.50 D steeper than the lower K in this case?**

Given K readings of 44.50/45.50, you would pick a lens with a curvature of 45.00 D (i.e., 0.50 D greater than the lower K, which is 44.50).

(c) **Why is the fit of rigid contact lenses always relative to the lower K?**

The base curve is always relative to the lower K because the flatter part of the cornea will support the rigid lens, while the steeper part of the cornea will drop away from the lens. Think of a round snow saucer sitting upside down (convex side up) on the very top of a hill that is steeper front-to-back than it is side-to-side. The side-to-side edges of the snow saucer will rest securely on the less steep (i.e., flattest) sides, while the steeper part of the hill will drop out from under the saucer.

(d) **Do you need to adjust the power of the contact lens based on how it is fit and, if so, how?**

Yes. Steeper Add Minus, Flatter Add Plus (SAM FAP).

When you select a K that is steeper than the lower K, tears will fill the gap between the cornea and lens, creating a "tear lens." Like any other lens, the tear lens has power: the power of the contact lens must be adjusted to compensate. Fitting a lens steeper will add plus power so you must add minus to the power that is ground into the contact lens, while fitting a lens flatter will add minus power so you must add plus power to the contact lens power. The mnemonic *SAM-FAP (steeper add minus, flatter add plus)* refers to how you adjust the power of the contact lens (Fig. 13.1).

Rigid contact lens fitting

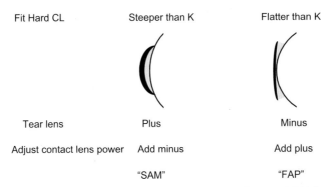

Fig. 13.1   How to adjust rigid contact lens power based on fit, "Steeper Add Minus, Flatter Add Plus" (SAM FAP).

6. **You fit Mr. Luddite with rigid gas permeable lenses, but he returns complaining that the lenses are uncomfortable, and that the whole world is going to fall apart if people can't even fit contact lenses like they used to. How would you assess the fit of the lenses? If there is "apical touch," what does that mean and how would you adjust the lenses?**

Apical touch → lens too loose → decrease radius of curvature or increase diameter of the lenses.

For rigid contact lenses, apply fluorescein and assess the pattern. A fit that is too tight (too steep) shows excessive apical clearance (bright green area centrally), while a lens that is too loose (too flat) shows minimal apical clearance (apical touch with no green area centrally). To adjust the fit, you can change the base curve or the diameter of the contact lens. Changing the base curve changes the radius of curvature; a shorter radius of curvature corresponds with a steeper curve, while a longer radius corresponds with a flatter curve. So, if the lens is:

Too tight → increase radius of curvature (lens too steep; higher radius = flatter lens)
Too loose → decrease the radius of curvature (lens too flat; lower radius = steeper lens)

You can also change the fit by changing the lens diameter. A smaller diameter will fit more loosely (consider that an infinitely small diameter would be like a flat surface that would move more freely around the eye) while a larger diameter will fit more snugly (imagine a suction cup sticking onto the eye). So, if the lens is:

Too tight → decrease the diameter of the lens
Too loose → increase the diameter of the lens

In this case you find that the lens has apical touch and you decrease the radius of curvature. Mr. Luddite's comfort is improved with the new lenses and he mails a typewritten letter to your office endorsing your skills.

7. **The K-readings of a prospective contact lens wearer are 42.50/44.75 @ 85. Refraction gives 20/15 visual acuity with −3.50 sphere spectacle correction. Since he has**

2.25 D of corneal cylinder, should you prescribe a rigid or soft lens? Should the lens be spherical or toric?

A spherical soft lens is probably the best choice.

The only way to explain how a patient with this degree of corneal cylinder could have a spherical refraction is that there is lenticular cylinder that happens to compensate. This is sometimes referred to as "favorable" or "complementary" lenticular astigmatism. A spherical rigid lens is the worst choice, since it corrects the corneal cylinder and will unmask the complementary lenticular cylinder, leaving the patient with a large uncorrected astigmatic error. Try a spherical soft lens first, since it will not change the corneal cylinder and it is less expensive than a toric lens. If the spherical soft lens somehow changes the balance between corneal and lenticular astigmatism, you may have to use a toric soft contact lens to correct any residual astigmatism.

8. **An aphakic man wearing +12.00 D contact lenses requests glasses for backup.**

   (a) **What power spectacle is required, if the vertex distance of the new glasses will be 10 mm?**

   +10.75 D.

   This is a classic vertex distance question. First, locate the far point of the eye. The secondary focal point of the corrective lens should match the far point of the eye. In this case, the far point is 1/12 D = 0.083 m = 83 mm from the cornea. The man has hyperopia, so the far point is 83 mm *behind* the cornea. The new lens should have a secondary focal point that matches the far point of the eye. The location of the new lens is 10 mm in front of the cornea, which is 93 mm from the far point. The power, then, will be 1/0.093 m = +10.75 D (Fig. 13.2).

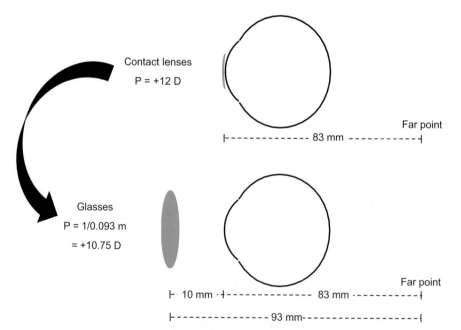

Fig. 13.2   Vertex distance change from contact lenses to glasses in hyperopia.

(b) **What power would be required for a woman wearing −12.00 D contact lenses who needs glasses (vertex distance 10 mm)?**

−13.75 D.

For the woman with myopia, the far point is 83 mm *in front* of the cornea, or (83 − 10) = 73 mm from the spectacle plane, so the power would be 1/0.073 = −13.7 D → Rx = −13.75 D (Fig. 13.3).

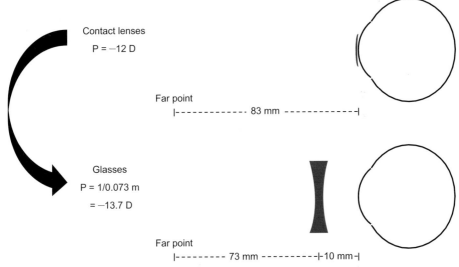

Contact lenses

P = −12 D

Far point
|------------- 83 mm -------------|

Glasses

P = 1/0.073 m

= −13.7 D

Far point
|--------- 73 mm ----------|-10 mm-|

Fig. 13.3 Vertex distance change from contact lenses to glasses in myopia.

9. **Anakin Koenia reports eye strain and diplopia while wearing his new glasses of −8 D OD and −3 D OS. Could switching to contact lenses improve the symptoms? Why?**

Yes, contact lenses reduce aniseikonia from anisometropia.

If the eyes have significantly different refractive error (anisometropia), spectacle correction creates retinal images of unequal size (i.e., aniseikonia; see Chapter 7, Refraction and Optical Dispensing). When the difference in spectacle power is greater than about 3 D, this can cause eye strain, headaches, and diplopia. Switching to contact lenses creates retinal images that are of almost equal size, relieving symptoms of aniseikonia (in both hyperopia and myopia).

10. **Will switching to contact lenses affect Anakin's accommodative demand? Would it be different if he had hyperopia?**

Yes, switching to contact lenses increases accommodative demand in myopia (in contrast, switching to contact lenses decreases accommodative demand in hyperopia).

The effect on accommodation depends on the underlying refractive error:
  - In *myopia*, switching from glasses to contact lenses increases accommodative demand. This is something to consider when switching a middle-aged patient

with myopia from glasses to contact lenses (or performing refractive surgery). The increased accommodative demand may precipitate symptoms of presbyopia.

- In *hyperopia*, switching from glasses to contact lenses decreases accommodative demand.

11. **Henry Hightower, a mechanical engineer, requires a toric soft contact lens for best vision. You prescribe −3.00 +1.00 × 90. Henry pulls out his phone to review the contact lens specifications available online, and he is skeptical about how the design will prevent a round lens from rotating and changing the axis. What possible mechanisms are there?**

There are three mechanisms that can be used to prevent the rotation of soft toric lenses:

1. *Adding prism ballast*: extra lens at the bottom, weight maintains alignment
2. *Creating thin zones*: at top and bottom, eyelid pressure maintains alignment
3. *Truncating bottom of lens*: straight edge aligns with lower eyelid

CHAPTER 14

Intraocular Lenses

1. **Name the two categories of formulas in common use for the calculation of intraocular lens (IOL) power. Give an example of each type.**

   1. *Regression formulas:* Empiric formulas derived by regression analysis of large numbers of clinical results (e.g., Sanders, Retzlaff, and Kraft [SRK], SRK II). Formulas based on artificial intelligence (AI) are a new and fancy version of an empiric formula based on results from many patients (though they use deep learning and not classic mathematical regression).
   2. *Theoretical formulas:* These are derived using principles of geometric optics, the basis of which is the Gullstrand model eye. Theoretical formulas (e.g., SRK-T, Holladay, Hoffer-Q, Haigis, Barrett True K) are more accurate and have for the most part replaced regression formulas, though AI-based formulas, e.g., the Hill-RBF (radial basis function) calculator are ascending.

2. **What is the SRK formula? What information is needed to calculate IOL power using the SRK formula?**

   The SRK formula is an empiric IOL formula:

   $$\text{SRK formula: } P_{(IOL)} = A - 2.5\,L - 0.9\,K$$

   To calculate P (Power of the IOL in diopters [D] for emmetropia), you need:
   1. A = IOL-specific lens constant
   2. K = average central corneal refractive power in diopters
   3. L = axial length in millimeters

3. **Based on the SRK formula, which has a greater impact on IOL power, a 1 D mistake in the K reading or a 1-mm mistake in axial length? Is an error of 1 mm in axial length more impactful in short or long eyes?**

   A 1 = mm mistake in axial length has more impact; short eyes.

   Based on the SRK formula, a 1-mm mistake in axial length has almost 3× the effect on the IOL power (2.5 D) compared to a 1 D mistake in K readings (0.9 D).
   Although it cannot be seen from the SRK formula, the shorter the axial length, the closer the retina is to the lens, and the more impactful an error of 1 mm. For example, using theoretical formulas, the calculation error is 3.75 D/mm in a 20-mm eye, 2.35 D/mm in a 23.5-mm eye, and 1.75 D/mm in a 30-mm eye.

4. **Based on your SRK IOL calculation, you select a lens with a power of +21.50 D. Unfortunately, a fly lands on the lens just as it is being loaded into the inserter, and the only available replacement lenses have an A constant that is 3.00 greater than the lens you planned to use. What power IOL should you choose?**

> *+24.50 D lens.*

> If the A constant changes, you should change the IOL power by the same amount. For an increase of 3.00 in the A constant, you should increase the IOL power by 3.00 and use a +24.50 D lens.

EXAM PEARL

Although the SRK formula is no longer used clinically for IOL calculations, it is still useful in understanding the principles of IOL calculations (and for answering exam questions!). Some common exam questions (with worked-out examples above) include:
- If you have an IOL with a different A constant, how does that change your IOL choice?
- If you indent the cornea by 1 mm doing an A scan, how much will that affect postoperative refraction?
- If you change the axial length (e.g., scleral buckle) by 2 mm, how does that change refraction?

---

5. **What important variable (not represented explicitly in the SRK formula) do modern theoretical IOL formulas take into account? Why is it important?**

> *Estimated lens position (ELP) – It is important because it affects the effective power of the IOL.*

> ELP is the distance from the principal plane of the cornea to the principal plane of the implanted IOL (Fig. 14.1). Older formulas referred to ELP indirectly as "anterior chamber depth," and the A constant in the SRK formula correlates with ELP for that lens design. There are various methods of calculating ELP; these differ among formulas, but the more accurately a formula predicts ELP, the more accurate the formula will be overall. ELP is important because an IOL that sits more anteriorly will be further from the retina and have considerably more effective plus power (thus requiring an IOL with relatively lower power), while an IOL that sits more posteriorly is closer to the retina and will have less effective plus power (thus requiring an IOL with relatively higher power) (Fig. 14.1).

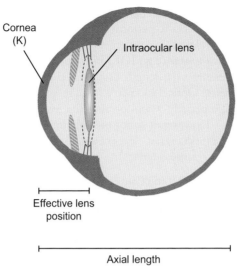

Fig. 14.1 Variables used in theoretical intraocular lens (IOL) formulas, including the effective lens position (ELP). If the ELP changes, the selected lens power will need to be adjusted opposite to the impact (e.g., lower-power IOL for anterior displacement).

6. How is corneal power measured? What are some common causes of errors?

Corneal power can be measured by keratometry (manual or automated) or by corneal topography/tomography.

Optical keratometers do not measure the refractive power of the cornea directly; they measure the *reflective* power of the anterior corneal surface. The instrument then infers the refractive corneal power by assuming all corneas have the same refractive index and the same relationship between the anterior and posterior corneal surfaces. Procedures that change the relationship between the anterior and posterior corneal surface (such as refractive surgery) or that change the refractive index of the cornea can cause a discrepancy between measured (inferred) corneal power and true corneal power.

Contact lenses, especially rigid contact lenses, change the shape of the cornea and can cause an incorrect K measurement. For this reason, contact lenses must be removed for a period of time prior to keratometry measurements. There is no universally accepted standard, but a contact-lens-free period of 1 week for soft contact lenses and 4 weeks for hard contact lenses is likely a safe recommendation for IOL calculations.

7. What are the two main methods used to measure the axial length of the eye? What are the advantages and disadvantages of each?

The two mechanisms for measuring axial length are ultrasonic and optical.

1. ***Ultrasonic measurement*** (known as A-scan ultrasonography) measures the time required for a sound pulse to travel from the cornea to the retina and back. The greater the distance, the longer it takes for the round trip. A-scans

can be performed using applanation (contact) or immersion (noncontact). Applanation is easier to perform than immersion but is prone to artificially shortened axial length measurements due to corneal indentation.

2. **Optical measurement** (e.g., IOLMaster optical biometer) uses an infrared laser to measure axial length using a technique called partial coherence interferometry. Optical biometry is more accurate and reproducible than ultrasound, especially when locating the fovea is an issue (e.g., posterior staphyloma). However, it is not possible to use this approach if fixation is poor or if the media is not clear enough for light transmission (e.g., squirming children or dense cataracts).

8. **You are about to perform cataract surgery, but you realize that the axial length seems high at 28 mm. Is there something you can quickly check to help determine if there was a measurement error in that eye?**

Check the axial length in the other eye and the refraction of both eyes.

The axial length is usually measured in both eyes and should be close to equal (unless there is a reason, such as a scleral buckle, anisometropia, or congenital eye disease). If there is an unexplained discrepancy, postpone the surgery to remeasure the axial length before proceeding. For a very long eye, the refraction would likely be myopic. If the patient has emmetropia or hyperopia, an error should be suspected.

9. **Should emmetropia be the goal in all cataract surgery? Give examples of when another target may be desirable.**

Most cataract surgeries aim for emmetropia. However, there are important exceptions:

- *To avoid anisometropia*: If the cataract is unilateral and the other eye has refractive error with no prospect of cataract surgery in the foreseeable future, then the target should be within about 3 D of the other eye to avoid intolerable aniseikonia.
- *Reading vision*: Patients with myopia may wish to remain at least somewhat myopic to allow for continued reading without glasses.
- *Post refractive surgery*: Although modern formulas are quite accurate, it may be desirable to aim for mild myopia if a patient has previously had refractive surgery for myopia to avoid a hyperopic surprise (see Question 10).

10. **Fay Coe previously had LASIK for myopia and now has cataracts. If you use manual keratometry and an older IOL formula, what postoperative refraction are you likely to get? What are three reasons why this occurs? What methods are available to avoid this error?**

A hyperopic surprise (which will be very annoying for you and for Fay) is most likely.

There are three reasons why IOL power may be underestimated after refractive surgery:

1. **Instrument error:** Keratometers and corneal topographers often miss the central zone flattened by myopic LASIK. As such, the anterior corneal power is overestimated and IOL power is underestimated.

2. *Error in assumed index of refraction:* The standardized refractive index used in optical keratometry considers both the refractive index of the cornea and the assumed posterior corneal curvature. Reduction in the anterior curvature of the cornea after refractive surgery leads to underestimation of the true negative posterior corneal power and consequent overestimation of the overall corneal refractive power. IOL power is therefore underestimated.

3. *Effective lens position:* Formulas that use axial length and keratometry to estimate the effective lens position of the IOL do not consider flattening of the cornea. As such, the formula incorrectly assumes that the lens will sit more anteriorly than it does. An IOL that is more posterior than expected will have less effective plus power.

All three errors lead to an underestimation of the power of IOL needed for emmetropia, leading to a hyperopic surprise. In the past, there were various ways to adjust IOL calculations after refractive surgery (e.g., clinical history method, contact lens method). However, more recently developed formulas (e.g., Barrett True K formula) have been shown to be quite accurate and do not require prerefractive surgery measurements.

11. **You are performing cataract surgery on Matt Ticulous, a successful malpractice attorney. After flawless phacoemulsification in record time, you load a +19.00 D lens into an injector and prepare to insert the lens in the capsular bag. To your horror, you realize that your new technician calculated the power for 1 D of HYPERopia, not the 1 D of MYopia that you requested. Your IOL power calculation computer is 30 miles away at your office, which is closed.**

   (a) **What power IOL do you insert in its place?**

   21.50 or 22.00 D IOL.

   The general rule of thumb for normally sized eyes is to change the calculated IOL power by 1.25 to 1.50 D for each diopter of desired ametropia. Therefore to go from a target of 1 D of hyperopia to 1 D of myopia (i.e., 2 D change in postoperative refraction), you need to add $2 \times 1.25 = 2.50$ D or $2 \times 1.50 = 3.00$ D of power to the IOL. As such, instead of a 19.00 IOL, you should select a +21.50 D or +22.00 D lens to aim for 1 D of myopia.

   (b) **You are about to insert a +21.50 D lens when you realize that the capsular bag has ruptured. You decide to place the lens in the sulcus. Should you change the lens power again? Why, in what direction (more or less power), and by how much? If you had to use an anterior chamber IOL, how much (approximately) and in what direction (higher or lower) should you change the power?**

   Yes. Less power; 1.0 D less for a sulcus lens and about 3.0 D less for an anterior chamber lens.

   You must decrease the power of the IOL. This is because the lens will sit more anteriorly and therefore will have more effective plus power. The amount of decrease depends on the power of the IOL (Table 14.1).

TABLE 14.1 ■ Adjustment of Intraocular Lens Power for Sulcus Placement

Bag Power	Sulcus Power
≤ +9.00 D	No change
+9.50 to +17.00 D	Decrease by 0.5 D
+17.50 to +28.00 D	Decrease by 1.0 D
> +28.00 D	Decrease by 1.5 D

For an anterior chamber IOL, the lens is located even more anteriorly, so you must decrease the power by a greater amount, generally about 3.0 D.

(c) **The postoperative course is rocky, and Mr. Ticulous returns for his 23rd postoperative visit, 6 months following the first cataract extraction. He notes decreased visual acuity in the pseudophakic eye. Best corrected visual acuity has dropped from 20/25 to 20/40. He also notes glare. How do you proceed?**

First, recheck the refraction, and check pinhole acuity with best correction in place. Evaluate the retinoscopic reflex to identify irregularities or opacities in the media. Look at the IOL position before dilating the pupil. Are possible sources of glare visible (e.g., IOL defects or an IOL edge)? Is there posterior capsule opacification? Corneal decompensation? Dilate the pupil and look again at the IOL and posterior capsule. If the front of the eye cannot explain the decrease in visual acuity, direct your attention to the retina and beyond.

(d) **Mr. Ticulous returns to you for surgery on the other eye. Sadly, the surgery went poorly, and it was not possible to place any lens at all. What should you do now?**

Contact lens or secondary IOL.

With monocular aphakia, glasses are likely not a good option (especially in adults), since aphakic spectacles are high plus (around +12 D), and the large amount of anisometropia will cause aniseikonia. A nonsurgical option would be to use a contact lens in the aphakic eye, which will correct the high hyperopia without inducing severe aniseikonia. In the long term, a secondary IOL will likely be the best solution for the patient.

12. **Mac Uloff has silicone oil in his eye and a cataract following a vitrectomy. What error will occur if you use standard ultrasonic biometry for IOL calculations? Why? How should you adjust the IOL power if the silicone oil will not be removed?**

If you use standard ultrasonic biometry, the axial length will be incorrectly too long. This is because sound travels considerably slower through silicone (980 m/s) than through vitreous (1532 m/s), so it takes longer for the sound to return, and the machine calculates an incorrectly long axial length. This would lead to an incorrectly low-power IOL and a hyperopic surprise. The error can be minimized by adjusting the settings on the A scan ultrasound or by using optical biometry.

Silicone oil has a refractive index that is higher than that of vitreous. If the silicone oil is left in place, the power of the posterior surface of the IOL will be decreased because the difference in refractive indices across this refractive surface is reduced (see Chapter 5, The Model Eye). The effective IOL power will therefore be less than expected. The power of the IOL should be increased by 3 to 5 D to compensate.

13. Mike Iddy is a 2-year-old child with a dense unilateral traumatic cataract following a fight with his brother.

   (a) How would you perform keratometry and biometry? If you aim for plano, what refractive error is likely to develop over the long term?

     Keratometry and immersion A scan under general anesthesia; aiming for plano will likely lead to myopia over the long term.

     For young children, keratometry and biometry are usually performed under general anesthesia just prior to surgery. Biometry will likely require ultrasonic measurement (ideally immersion A scan), as an optical measurement may not be able to penetrate the dense cataract and the child cannot fixate under anesthesia.

     Most children have a myopic shift over time as their eyes grow, so aiming for plano at this age will likely lead to long-term myopia. Most pediatric cataract surgeons aim for mild-to-moderate hyperopia in young children, depending on age.

   (b) Mike has 5 D of corneal astigmatism and his brother, Efren, who also has a unilateral traumatic cataract from the same unfortunate incident, has 5 D of lenticular astigmatism. Who would be most likely to benefit from a toric IOL? Why?

     Mike. Toric IOLs correct for corneal astigmatism.

     Toric IOLs correct corneal astigmatism, so Mike would benefit. Lenticular astigmatism is not relevant, since the crystalline lens will be removed.

14. Dr. Amy B. Dextrous, a practicing neurosurgeon, would like to be glasses-free post cataract surgery. What options do you have?

While no surgery is guaranteed to eliminate glasses in all situations, there are several options for patients who would like to decrease their dependence on glasses:

   1. *Monovision.* Aim for distance vision in one eye and near vision in the other. This might not be acceptable to a neurosurgeon who requires precise binocularity working with an operating microscope and is generally not recommended for patients with significant phorias, as it may precipitate decompensation of the strabismus.

   2. *Multifocal IOLs.* Again, this may not work, as some patients (especially those who are fastidious) cannot tolerate the reduced contrast sensitivity inherent in the design of any multifocal IOL.

   3. *Accommodating IOLs.* These lenses are designed to change their effective lens position when the ciliary muscle relaxes and contracts, such that the IOL

moves forward in the accommodative state. Current designs generate only small amounts of accommodative power.

In this case a long discussion may be warranted to balance patient expectations with what can be accomplished with surgery. For example, perhaps the patient would accept monovision at home, understanding that spectacles or contact lenses would still be needed at work.

15. What are the two main types of multifocal lenses and how do they work? How do multifocal lenses affect depth of focus and contrast sensitivity?

Multiple-zone refractive IOLs and diffractive multifocal IOLs; increase depth of focus and reduce contrast sensitivity.

Multiple-zone refractive IOLs use concentric rings with different powers (Fig. 14.2). *Diffractive multifocal IOLs* use an overall spherical shape for distance vision, with a stepped structure on the posterior (or sometimes anterior) surface. Diffraction from the diffractive surface creates a second image from constructive interference (Fig. 14.3).

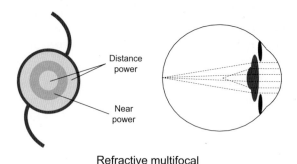

Refractive multifocal
intraocular lens

Fig. 14.2   Refractive intraocular lens design: concentric rings have different refractive powers.

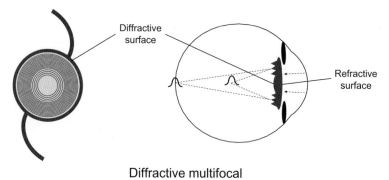

Diffractive multifocal
intraocular lens

Fig. 14.3   Diffractive intraocular lens design: diffractive surface on the posterior surface of the lens.

By definition, multifocal lenses increase the depth of focus. However, by splitting the amount of light entering the eye, there is an inevitable loss of contrast sensitivity. As such, patients with poor contrast sensitivity function (e.g., retinal dystrophies, macular disease) are generally poor candidates for multifocal IOLs.

CHAPTER 15

Refractive Surgery

1. **What is the shape of the normal cornea: oblate or prolate? Does the cornea have positive or negative spherical aberration?**

   Prolate; positive spherical aberration.

   The normal cornea is prolate. This means that it is steepest in the center and flattens toward the periphery. This acts to counteract the spherical aberration of the lens, which has its highest refractive power in the periphery. However, the magnitude of the prolate contour is not enough to completely neutralize spherical aberration, so the cornea (and the eye) still has positive spherical aberration.

2. **How does refractive surgery on the cornea correct myopia? What is the basic principle conceptually, and how is it expressed mathematically?**

   In myopia, there is too much refractive power for the axial length of the eye. In refractive surgery for myopia, the cornea is flattened in the region where traversing light will enter the pupil. Flattening the cornea increases r, the radius of curvature of the cornea. This decreases the refractive power of the cornea, P, as per the equation for the refracting power of a spherical refracting surface (see Chapter 2, Vergence, Lenses, Objects, and Images):

$$P = \frac{(n' - n)}{r}$$

3. **How does hyperopic refractive surgery work?**

   In hyperopia, the cornea is not strong enough for a given axial length, so the procedure must somehow increase the central corneal curvature (where it overlies the pupil). This can be accomplished with excimer laser sculpting or by using conductive keratoplasty to "cook" the corneal periphery, thus creating a band of flat, shrunken cornea peripherally that causes compensatory steepening centrally.

4. **How can laser ablation of the cornea be used to correct astigmatism? If keratometry suggests that the 45-degree meridian is steepest, what sort of ablation would be performed?**

   The key to correcting astigmatism is to alter the cornea in an elliptical pattern that is complementary to the existing astigmatism. One way to achieve this is to flatten the cornea preferentially in the steepest meridian. For this patient, an elliptical ablation would need to take place in the 45-degree meridian to flatten the cornea more along this meridian.

5. **A 42-year-old man with a refraction of −5.00 +0.75 × 90 in both eyes presents for LASIK. He is a major donor to your nonprofit foundation, and he wants to have the procedure tomorrow, in time for a family reunion. He is looking forward to many years of independence from glasses. What are the relative and absolute contraindications to LASIK in general? What aspects of the history or physical examination would reduce your enthusiasm for moving forward in this case?**

There are several relative and absolute contraindications to LASIK and related forms of refractive surgery. These include:
- Unrealistic expectations
- Refractive concerns
  - Changing refraction (must be stable within 0.5 diopters [D] for 1 year)
  - Very high degrees of myopia, hyperopia, or astigmatism
    - The US FDA allows for myopia up to 12 D, astigmatism up to 6 D, and hyperopia up to 6 D, but many surgeons do not go this far
- Ocular conditions
  - Ocular surface disease
    - Dry eye disease
    - Uncontrolled blepharitis
    - Epithelial basement membrane dystrophy
    - Irregular astigmatism
  - Thin cornea/corneal ectasia
    - Keratoconus (including form fruste)
    - Pellucid marginal degeneration
    - Any other cause of corneal ectasia; need to review topography
  - Fuchs endothelial dystrophy
  - Highly myopic eyes with untreated peripheral retinal tears (suction ring during LASIK could exacerbate)
  - Strabismus; while not a contraindication, strabismus can worsen after refractive surgery, especially if the target is monovision or if myopia is overcorrected
- Systemic contraindications:
  - Autoimmune disease
  - Pregnancy or lactation (refraction may be unstable)
  - Plan for isotretinoin treatment (will cause dry eye)

In this case, the patient is in the prepresbyopic years and may end up requiring reading glasses after LASIK, so his expectations of being independent of glasses for many years are unrealistic.

6. **Bill D. Bridges is a mechanical engineer who comes to your clinic for "bladeless" LASIK. He says that he will only consider all-laser surgery and would like to know which types of lasers you will use and the underlying mechanisms. Without even looking at your beloved copy of *Last-Minute Optics* (Third Edition), you state that there are two types of lasers used to perform refractive surgery:**

1. *Excimer laser.* The excimer laser performs the corneal ablation. The mechanism is photoablation, in which wavelengths in the UV range are used to break covalent chemical bonds.
2. *Femtosecond laser.* The femtosecond laser makes the corneal flap. The mechanism is plasma-induced ablation. The laser strips electrons from atoms, which

leads to plasma formation and allows for a well-defined removal of corneal tissue without thermal damage. The femtosecond laser is the technology behind small-incision lenticule extraction (SMILE) surgery.

7. **Are there limits to how steep or flat the cornea should be after refractive surgery?**

   Yes.

   Excessively flat or steep corneal curvature can increase aberrations and decrease vision quality. As such, it is advisable to avoid postop corneal curvature less than 33 D or greater than 50 D.

8. **What problems may occur with a small ablation zone or large pupil?**

   If the pupil is large (>8 mm) or the ablation zone is small (≤6 mm), the edge of the ablation zone may be within the entrance to the pupil of the eye. Diffraction at the edge of the "aperture" can increase spherical aberration and cause glare, starbursts, halos, and poor-quality vision, especially at night. In addition, the edge will create two refractive domains within the pupil, which may lead to multifocal optics and monocular diplopia (even triplopia in some cases). Modern algorithms use larger ablation zones and transition zones to try to minimize the risk and severity of these problems.

9. **Mr. Lee Tigious presents to you seeking laser vision correction, but he has been told that he has "the stigmatism" and he worries that it is an incurable disease. Refraction is:**

   OD: −3.75 +1.25 × 90 → 20/15
   OS: −3.75 +1.25 × 90 → 20/15

   Keratometry measures:

   OD: 45.00 @ 90/46.00 @ 180
   OS: 45.00 @ 90/46.00 @ 180

   What kind of astigmatism does he have? Is the astigmatism going to be a problem in this case?

   Compound myopic astigmatism and with-the-rule astigmatism; he has complementary lenticular astigmatism that can be corrected with creative refractive surgery, but this may complicate future cataract surgery.

   In this case, the power cross places −3.75 D on the 90-degree meridian and −2.50 D on the 180-degree meridian. Both numbers are negative, so this is compound myopic astigmatism. The axis of plus (correcting) cylinder is at 90 degrees, so it is with-the-rule astigmatism.

   The keratometry results indicate that there is 1 D of corneal astigmatism, so this seems at first glance to correspond roughly with the refraction. But does it? The cornea is steeper in the 180-degree meridian. This would be corrected by providing about a diopter of plus power in the 90-degree meridian, plus cylinder axis 180. That is, given these keratometry measurements, you should expect the corrective lenses to be "(some sphere) +1.00 × 180." You have uncovered a rare case of corneal astigmatism that is neutralized (and then overcompensated for) by complementary lenticular astigmatism. If your refractive surgery eliminates the corneal astigmatism, the patient will end up with over 2 D of uncorrected lenticular astigmatism.

Since refractive surgery is generally based on the subjective refraction, the lenticular astigmatism should not be a problem. He therefore may have refractive surgery, but the corneal astigmatism should be left as is (thus requiring +1.25 of astigmatic correction at 90 degrees for best vision postoperatively) or the corneal astigmatism should be *increased* to fully mask the lenticular astigmatism. However, should the patient ever need cataract surgery, the complementary lenticular astigmatism will be removed, and a toric intraocular lens will then be advisable to replace the lenticular astigmatism and balance the corneal astigmatism.

10. **After LASIK, a patient complains that something is off with his vision. Uncorrected visual acuity is 20/25+ and the refraction is +2.00−4.00 × 65 in the left eye. The right eye is doing well. What is the likely cause? How could you confirm this?**

Irregular astigmatism.

The refraction (with 4 D of astigmatism) is not consistent with an uncorrected visual acuity of 20/25+; that is, the uncorrected vision is too good for a patient with that much *regular* astigmatism. A post-LASIK refraction that is inconsistent with visual acuity is most likely due to *irregular* astigmatism secondary to faulty ablation. To confirm this, irregular astigmatism can be detected as scissoring on streak retinoscopy, improved vision with a rigid contact lens, irregularity on corneal topography, or wavefront analysis.

11. **What is wavefront analysis and how is it performed? What is the potential benefit of using wavefront-guided ablation?**

Wavefront analysis is a method of describing irregular astigmatism quantitatively. One method of performing wavefront analysis is to use a Hartmann-Shack aberrometer. With the Hartmann-Shack aberrometer, a low-intensity laser acts as a point source of light reflecting back out through the pupil. A Hartmann screen is placed in front of the eye and small apertures isolate narrow beams of light. The isolated light beams then strike a sensor that measures where the light rays are dispersed compared to where they should have been with a wavefront from a perfect optical system (Fig. 15.1).

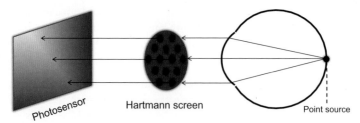

Fig. 15.1 Hartmann-Shack aberrometer.

Wavefront-guided ablation uses the patient's wavefront analysis to try to minimize the induction of higher-order aberrations. When successful, this improves vision quality overall and night vision in particular.

CHAPTER 16

Prisms and Diplopia

1. **Parallel light passes through a base-down prism with a power of 10 prism diopters (PD or Δ). In which direction is the light bent? At 1 m from the prism, how far is the light displaced? What about at 2 m and 3 m?**

   Light bends toward the base; light is displaced 10 cm at 1 m, 20 cm at 2 m, and 30 cm at 3 m.

   A prism bends light toward the base (remember **BB** → **B**ends toward the **B**ase). The definition of a PD is a displacement of 1 cm at 1 m. That is, a 1 PD prism would deviate light 1 cm at 1 m. Therefore a 10 PD prism deviates light 10 cm at 1 m. The light is deviated in a linear fashion, so that at 2 m the light is deviated $2 \times 10 = 20$ cm, and at 3 m, the light is deviated $3 \times 10 = 30$ cm (Fig. 16.1).

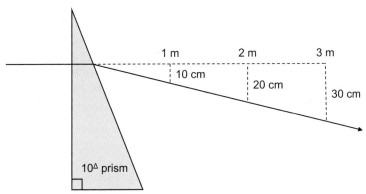

Fig. 16.1 Deviation of light at 1 m, 2 m, and 3 m by a 10^Δ prism.

EXAM PEARL

Be careful not to confuse prism diopters (PD or Δ) with diopters (D). Despite the similar sounding names, these are completely different units.

PD or Δ: A prism diopter is defined as a 1-cm displacement of light at a distance of 1 m from a prism. It is used to describe the strength of prisms and the magnitude of strabismus.

D: A diopter describes the vergence of light or the power of a lens or mirror. It is the inverse of meters, $D = m^{-1}$ (which is why you are constantly taking reciprocals to go from distance to diopters and back again).

2. Calculate the prismatic displacement at positions A through E (Fig. 16.2).

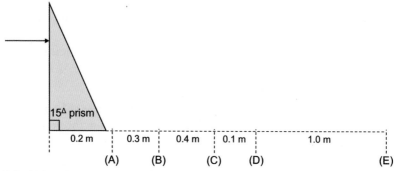

Fig. 16.2   Light displacement by 15△ prism. (Prism should be considered to be infinitely thin.)

The light ray will be displaced (in a linear fashion) 15 cm toward the prism base for each 1 m traveled.
(A) 3 cm (= 15 PD * 0.2 m)
(B) 7.5 cm (= 15 PD * (0.2 + 0.3) m)
(C) 13.5 cm (= 15 PD * (0.2 + 0.3 + 0.4) m)
(D) 15 cm (= 15 PD * 1 m)
(E) 30 cm (= 15 PD * 2 m)

3. During an optics review, an ancient professor uses an old-fashioned movie projector to share a documentary about the making of the second edition of an excellent optics review book. A student, Bard tuTeers, happens to be sitting close to the projector, which is 6 m from the screen. Bard places a 10 PD prism base down in front of the projector.

(a) Which way does the image of the projected slide move? How far does it move?

The image moves down 60 cm.

The light from the projector bends toward the base. As such, the image moves down (Fig. 16.3). We know from the definition of a PD that the image will be displaced 10 cm at a distance of 100 cm (1 m). Since the screen is six times that far away (6 m), we simply multiply 10 cm by 6 to get 60 cm. More formally:

$$\text{Displacement of the image DI (in cm)} = \text{power of prism (PD)} \times \text{distance (m)}$$
$$DI = 10\Delta \times 6 \text{ m}$$
$$DI = 60 \text{ cm}$$

(b) Is the image real or virtual?

Real.

This is a *real image*. It is on the same side of the prism as the light rays that define it (i.e., not located by imaginary extensions of light rays).

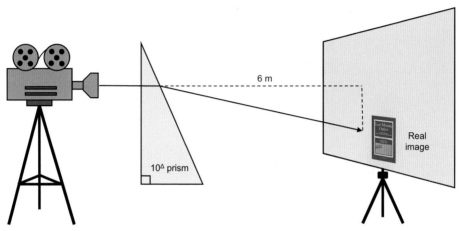

Fig. 16.3   When the prism is placed in front of the projector, the real image (light from projector) is displaced toward the prism base by 60 cm on the screen (screen does not move).

4. **Bard eventually gets bored to tears with this trick, so now he takes the 10 PD prism away from the projector and looks at the screen through the prism, still with the base down. In which direction does the image of the book cover appear to move? What about the image of the screen? Is this a real or virtual image?**

The book appears to move up toward the apex of the prism; the screen appears to move up as well; virtual image.

Note that at first, this seems opposite to the situation in Question 3. In both cases, a base-down prism is used. However, in the first case (prism in front of projector), the real image appears to move down, while in the second case (viewing the image through the prism), the virtual image appears to move up.

How can this be? The light is still bent toward the base, but the brain assumes that the light traveled along a straight path. As such, imaginary extensions of the rays of light (from both the image of the book and from the screen itself) must be drawn to determine the perceived image location, which is toward the prism apex (Fig. 16.4). Since imaginary extension lines must be drawn to locate the image, it is a virtual image.

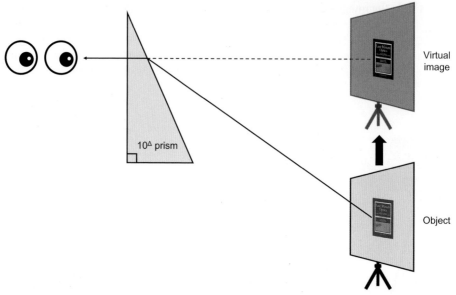

Fig. 16.4 When looking through a prism, the image is virtual and appears to be displaced toward the prism apex.

EXAM PEARL

It is easy to get confused with the images produced by prisms. Keep in mind that, in every case, light is bent toward the base of the prism. There are two common scenarios:
- The light rays that pass through the prism to the opposite side form a *real image* deviated toward the *base* (the projector scenario).
- If someone looks through the prism, imaginary lines must be drawn to the same side of the object that form a *virtual image* deviated toward the *apex* (the viewing scenario).

5. How do you find the optical center of an ordinary lens?

If you shine a laser through a lens, the light passing through the lens will experience prismatic displacement at almost any location on the lens except one. That point, where the laser passes through the lens without prismatic displacement, is known as the optical center.

Note that the optical center of a lens is not necessarily at its geometric center. The easiest way to find the optical center is to place it in a lensmeter and adjust the lens horizontally and vertically until the target is centered within the reticle of the eyepiece. Once identified, you can use the marking tool in the lensmeter to mark the location.

6. What is Prentice's rule?

Prentice's rule defines the prismatic effect of lenses (Fig. 16.5). Prentice's rule determines the induced prismatic power of a lens when light passes through a point at a given distance from the optical center. The orientation of prismatic power is specified by the direction of the base (by convention). A vertical prism is described as base up or base down. A horizontal prism is described as base in or base out.

$$\Delta = h \times P$$

Δ – Prism (in prism diopters)

h – Distance from optical center (in cm)

P – Power of the lens (in diopters)

Fig. 16.5 Prentice's rule.

EXAM PEARL

Prentice's rule is one of the only formulas that uses a distance in cm (rather than m). Therefore the distance from the optical center must always be converted to cm before the induced prismatic power is calculated.

7. **How do you determine the direction a light ray is displaced when it passes through a lens?**

Light is displaced toward the base of the induced prism. The orientation of the prism base depends on whether the lens is a plus or minus lens, as well as whether the light passes above, below, right, or left of the optical center.

For a plus lens, light experiences base-down prism when it passes above the optical center, and base-up prism when it passes below the optical center. For a minus lens, the opposite is true: base-up when above the optical center and base-down when below the optical center (Fig. 16.6).

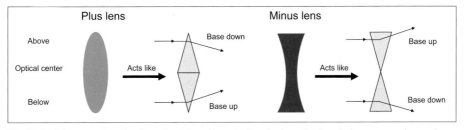

Fig. 16.6 Diagram showing how to determine whether induced prism is base up or base down depending on the type of lens (plus/minus) and whether light passes above or below the optical center.

For a plus lens, light experiences base-in prism when it passes temporal to the optical center, and base-out prism when it passes nasal to the optical center. For a minus lens, light experiences base-in when it passes nasal to the optical center, and base-out when it passes temporal to the optical center.

EXAM PEARL

To remember which way the light deviated by a lens, we constructed a visual mnemonic. A plus lens in profile looks very much like two prisms base-to-base; a minus lens in profile looks very much like two prisms apex-to-apex (Fig. 16.6).

8. **Dee V. Eight picks up a –2 D trial lens and looks 1 cm below the optical center. What prismatic deviation is induced? What if Dee was looking 15 mm below the optical center of a +3 D lens?**

   2 PD base down; 4.5 PD base up.

   Use Prentice's rule to calculate the induced deviation (Fig. 16.7).

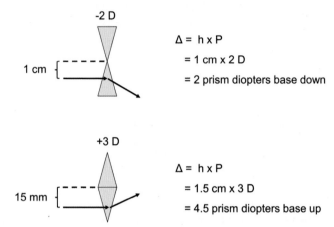

Fig. 16.7   Induced prism through a –2 D and +3 D lens.

9. **Tiffany Zale, a 20-year-old jewelry designer, is prescribed glasses due to contact lens intolerance. The prescription is –10 D sphere in both eyes. She reads 12.5 mm below the optical center of each lens.**

   (a) **What is the induced prism in the reading position in each eye?**

   12.5 PD base down.

   $$\Delta = h \times P$$
   $$= 1.25 \text{ cm} \times 10 \text{ D} (\text{remember to convert mm to cm!})$$
   $$= 12.5 \text{ prism diopters base down}$$

   (b) **How far would the image of a jewel held 0.5 m away appear to be displaced for each eye?**

   6.25 cm.

   $$\text{Displacement} = 12.5 \text{ PD} \times 0.5 \text{ m}$$
   $$= 6.25 \text{ cm}$$

(c) If Tiffany reached for the image of the jewel with forceps, would she reach above or below it?

Above.

Tiffany would reach for the image of the jewel that she sees. Since the image is displaced up (virtual image deviated toward the apex), she would reach above the actual object (Fig. 16.8).

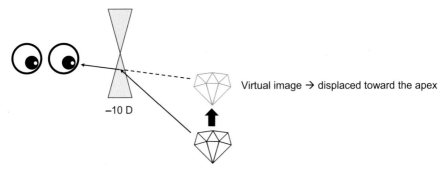

Fig. 16.8 Tiffany viewing a (virtual) image through induced base-down prism.

(d) Is the image seen by Tiffany real or virtual?

Virtual.

The image is located using imaginary extensions of the rays of light (Fig. 16.8).

10. **Devee Eiting has glasses of –8 D OD and –10 D OS.**

    (a) What is the net induced prism when Devee views an object 1 cm below the optical centers?

    2 PD base down on the left, or 2 PD base up on the right (Fig. 16.9).

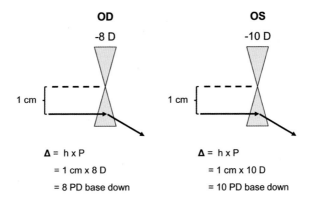

Net Δ = 2 PD base down OS or 2 PD base up OD

Fig. 16.9 Explanation of answer to Question 10(a). *OD,* Right eye; *OS,* left eye; *PD,* prism diopters.

(b) What is the induced prism looking 0.5 cm to the right of the optical centers?

1 PD base in Fig. 16.10.

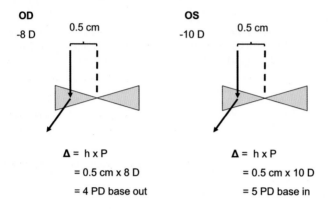

Δ = h x P

    = 0.5 cm x 8 D

    = 4 PD base out

Δ = h x P

    = 0.5 cm x 10 D

    = 5 PD base in

Net Δ = 1 PD base in

(In theory, you could also say 1 PD base left OD or 1 PD base right OS,

but we always use base in / out for horizontal prism by convention)

Fig. 16.10 Explanation of answer to Question 10(b). *OD*, Right eye; *OS*, left eye; *PD*, prism diopters.

(c) What is the induced prism with each eye converging 3 mm nasally?

5.4 PD base in Fig. 16.11.

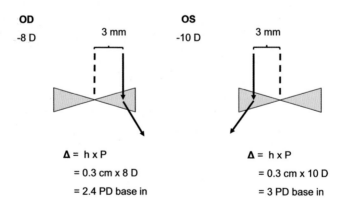

Δ = h x P

    = 0.3 cm x 8 D

    = 2.4 PD base in

Δ = h x P

    = 0.3 cm x 10 D

    = 3 PD base in

Net Δ = 5.4 PD base in

Fig. 16.11 Explanation of answer to Question 10(c). *OD*, Right eye; *OS*, left eye; *PD*, prism diopters.

11. Sal Linder is wearing glasses with a power of +2.00 –3.00 × 90 OD; –5.00 –2.00 × 180 OS.

    (a) What prism power does Sal experience when looking 2 cm below the optical center of the lenses?

    18 PD base-up OD or 18 PD base-down OS.

    The first step in solving a problem like this is to draw the power crosses of the spectacle lenses (Fig. 16.12).

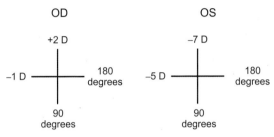

OD   OS

Fig. 16.12   Power crosses of Sal's glasses. *OD,* Right eye; *OS,* left eye.

    Then use the power in the vertical meridian for vertical displacement and the power in the horizontal meridian for horizontal displacement. In this case, when viewing 2 cm below the optical centers:

$$\text{OD: } \Delta = h \times P \qquad \text{OS: } \Delta = h \times P$$
$$= 2 \text{ cm} \times 2 \text{ D} \qquad\quad = 2 \text{ cm} \times 7 \text{ D}$$
$$= 4 \text{ PD base up} \qquad = 14 \text{ PD base down}$$

    The net prism is 18 PD base-up OD or 18 PD base-down OS.

    (b) What if Sal converges his eyes 1 cm nasal to the optical center of both lenses?

    6 PD base in.

    When viewing 1 cm nasal to the optical center through minus lens power, base-in prism is experienced by each eye (use the horizontal powers from the same power crosses in Fig. 16.12):

$$\text{OD: } \Delta = h \times P \qquad\qquad \text{OS: } \Delta = h \times P$$
$$= 1 \text{ cm} \times 1 \text{ D} \qquad\qquad = 1 \text{ cm} \times 5 \text{ D}$$
$$= 1 \text{ PD base in} \qquad\qquad = 5 \text{ PD base in}$$
$$\text{(nasal to optical center)} \qquad \text{(nasal to optical center)}$$

    The net prism is 6 PD base in.

EXAM PEARL

By convention, *prisms are always defined by the direction of base*. For prisms in glasses, we use base up and down for vertical prisms, and we use base in and out for horizontal prisms (instead of, say "base left" or "base right"). As a result, vertical and horizontal prisms combine differently when you need to calculate net prism:

1. **Net vertical prism**
   (a) Symmetric vertical prism cancels; for example, 6 PD base down in both eyes gives a net prism of 0, but image displacement will occur. (This is sometimes referred to as "yoked prism".)
   (b) Asymmetric vertical prism adds; for example, 6 PD base-down prism OD and 6 PD base-up prism OS gives a net of 12 PD base-down prism OD or 12 PD base-up prism OS (these are equivalent).

2. **Net horizontal prism**
   (a) Symmetric horizontal prism adds; for example, 6 PD base out in both eyes gives a net prism of 12 PD base out.
   (b) Asymmetric horizontal prism cancels; for example, 6 PD base-in prism OD, 6 PD base-out prism OS gives a net prism of 0, but image displacement will occur.

---

12. **Given that Sal experiences an induced prism of 18 PD base-up OD (or 18 PD base-down OS) looking 2 cm below the optical centers of the glasses:**

    (a) **What type of deviation is induced?**

    Right *hyper*tropia of 18 PD (or left *hypo*tropia of 18 PD)

    (b) **What prism could be used to correct the deviation?**

    18 PD base down over the right eye or 18 PD base up over the left (The correcting prism is the opposite of the induced prism)

13. **Given that Sal experiences an induced prism of 6 PD base in when looking 1 cm nasal to the optical centers of the glasses:**

    (a) **What type of deviation is induced?**

    Esotropia 6 PD

    (b) **What prism could be used to correct the deviation?**

    No prism is likely needed, since base-in prism helps with convergence, and the only reason Sal would be looking 1 cm nasal to the optical centers in both eyes would be because he was doing some near work. However, if for some reason prism was needed, the deviation would be neutralized by 6 PD base out over either eye.

EXAM PEARL

The induced strabismic deviation caused by a prism confuses many people (which makes it a great exam question!). There are several methods to try to remember what kind of deviation is induced by a given prism:

1. **Memorize**: The deviation is toward the *base* (e.g., *base-up* prism induces a *hypertropia*).

2. **Ray tracing**: Imagine a laser pointer inside the eye, projecting outward. The prism shifts the laser light toward the base. The line of sight will follow this same pathway. For example, a base-up prism will shift the line of sight upward, so the eye would be effectively hypertropic.

3. **Clinical experience**: Think about how you would neutralize the prism (e.g., a base-in prism would be neutralized by a base-out prism; since a base-out prism treats esotropia, the base-in prism must have induced an esotropia).

It is important to realize that an induced deviation does not mean that the eyes have physically moved. It just means that the line of sight has shifted relative to the target. For instance, if you use a base-in prism to induce an esotropia, the eyes have not moved inward. Instead, the "induced esotropia" refers to the fact that the prism has bent the light so that the eyes are now looking inward relative to the fixation target.

---

14. **Since Sal experiences an induced prism of 18 PD base-up OD (or 18 PD base-down OS), what fusional movements would be needed to regain fusion? What eye movements would be needed to regain fusion for an induced prism of 6 PD base in?**

   Induced prism 18 PD base-up OD → right hypertropia → right eye moves *down* 18 PD to fuse

   or

   Induced prism 18 PD base-down OS → left hypotropia → left eye moves *up* 18 PD to fuse (Good luck trying to fuse that much vertical prism! Most patients can fuse only 2–4 PD of vertical prism.)

   Induced prism 6 PD base in → esotropia 6 PD → eyes need to move *outward* (diverge) 6 PD to fuse for distance, but they are already converging so there is likely no need for any fusional vergence.

EXAM PEARL

It is important to differentiate a *prism-induced deviation* from the *fusional movements made to regain fusion*. We have seen people almost come to blows arguing over this point and found errors in some review manuals.

It is best to think of fusional movements as a completely separate process that some patients may be able to use to compensate for an induced deviation. For example, a base-out prism causes an exotropia on alternate cover testing of an orthophoric subject. Any inward movement of the eyes would only occur later, under binocular viewing conditions, after the subject had time to adapt to the prism, and only if they had binocular fusion as well as the capacity to overcome the induced deviation by converging.

15. **A 7 PD prism is placed base up-and-out in the 45-degree meridian over the left eye of a patient with orthotropia. The patient complains of diplopia.**

   (a) **What is the induced vertical prismatic power?**

   5 PD base-up OS.

   The first step for decoding an oblique prism problem is to break the prism down into its vertical and horizontal components. This requires a bit of high school trigonometry. Since the angle is 45 degrees, the two components are equal (Fig. 16.13).

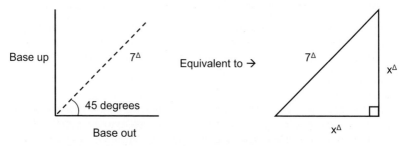

Fig. 16.13   7 prism diopters at 45 degrees, oriented base up and out.

   This calls for the Pythagorean theorem (little did you know while making paper airplanes in high school math class that you would one day be using the Pythagorean theorem to help people see better):

$$x^2 + x^2 = 7^2$$
$$2x^2 = 49$$
$$x^2 = 24.5 \, (\text{approximately } 25)$$
$$x = {\sim}5 \, \text{PD}$$

   The vertical component of induced prism power is thus 5 PD base up, oriented over the left eye.

   (b) **What is the horizontal component of the prism power?**

   5 PD base out (same reasoning as the previous answer).

   It may seem counterintuitive that you can get both 5 PD base up and 5 PD base out from a single 7 PD prism. Welcome to the magic of math and science.

   (c) **What types of strabismus appear to be present when an alternate cover test is performed?**

   Left hypertropia 5 PD and an exotropia 5 PD.

(d) What prism could you place over the right eye to eliminate the diplopia?

7 PD, base up and in.

To correct a left hypertropia (right hypotropia), a base-up prism is used over the right eye. To correct an exotropia, a base-in prism is used over either eye.

16. What are Fresnel prisms? What are their advantages and disadvantages versus conventional prisms?

Fresnel prisms are thin, plastic prisms that adhere to glasses via electrostatic attraction (no adhesive required). The prism effect is achieved by a series of small prisms at a given angle (Fig. 16.14). The prisms are cut to fit the back of a spectacle lens and are simply floated onto a small pool of water on the lens, then pressed on like a decal.

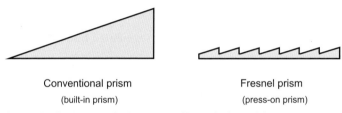

Conventional prism
(built-in prism)

Fresnel prism
(press-on prism)

Fig. 16.14   Conventional prism versus Fresnel prism of the same strength.

The advantages of Fresnel prisms are that they are thin, relatively inexpensive, and easy to use for short periods of time. However, they are visible to others, cause scattering of light at groove edges, and have an optical quality that is inferior to that of ground-in prisms. Fresnel prisms are particularly useful for transient deviations or as a trial before prescribing more expensive ground-in prism spectacles.

17. What are the indications to give spectacles with prisms? What types of strabismus are best treated with prisms?

There are several indications for prisms in spectacles:

- Restore binocularity for a patient with constant strabismus
- Ease asthenopia for a patient with phoria or intermittent tropia
- Perform prism adaptation to bring out the "true" amount of esotropia prior to surgery
- Preview the postoperative result of planned strabismus surgery
- Treat an anomalous head posture due to nystagmus with a null point or a hemifield defect (using yoked prisms)

Prisms work best for patients with small, comitant deviations. Larger deviations are harder to treat with prisms, simply because of the weight of and chromatic aberration produced by spectacle prisms. Consider a trial of Fresnel prisms before grinding the prism into the spectacle lens, but be aware that some patients cannot tolerate the glare and decreased visual acuity caused by a Fresnel prism.

18. How should prisms be written in prescriptions?

Always specify the *amount and direction of the base of the prism*, as well as the lens or lenses into which the prism should be incorporated. For larger comitant strabismus, it is best to split the prism, otherwise one lens will be very heavy compared with the other. For incomitant strabismus, it is best to try to place the prism over the eye with limited movements to bring the image to the eye, rather than requiring the oculomotor system to try to bring the eye to the image, which may induce a secondary deviation.

For combinations of horizontal and vertical prism, opticians are perfectly happy for you to write out the horizontal and vertical prism separately; they will then use that information to grind in the prism, with the net result being an oblique prism. However, if the goal is to apply a Fresnel press-on prism over one eye, then it is important to be exact about the direction (e.g., "6 PD base up and out in the 25-degree meridian of the left eye").

19. What are the two most common types of segmented bifocals and how do they differ?

There are two main types of segmented bifocals: *round-top* and *flat-top* (Fig. 16.15). Both provide extra plus power in the reading position. The main difference is the location of the optical center of the bifocal segment. In round-top bifocals, the optical center is at the bottom of the segment, while in flat-top bifocals, the optical center is near the top of the segment.

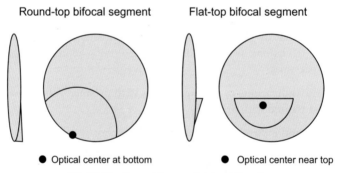

Round-top bifocal segment   Flat-top bifocal segment

● Optical center at bottom   ● Optical center near top

Fig. 16.15   Round-top vs. flat-top bifocals.

20. What are image jump and image displacement? How can these be minimized? Which type of bifocals are best for myopia and which are best for hyperopia?

Image jump is a *sudden* shift in the position of an image caused by prismatic power at the top of the bifocal segment. Image jump can be thought of as a dynamic phenomenon that occurs at the point of transition.

Image displacement is the *net shift* of an image produced by the total prismatic power acting in the reading position due to the combined effect of the glasses and bifocal segment. Image displacement can be thought of as a static phenomenon that occurs when the eyes have settled into the reading position.

Image jump is minimized by placing the optical center of the bifocal at the top of the segment so that there is no prismatic power at the point where the line of sight crosses into the bifocal power. This is best achieved with a flat-top bifocal design (as opposed to a round-top bifocal). There is also no image jump with progressive lenses or "executive" style bifocals (where the entire lower half of the lens has bifocal power and the upper and lower segments are bonded at their optical centers).

Image displacement is minimized by giving a bifocal segment with a prismatic effect that is opposite to the distance segment. For plus lenses (with a base-up effect when reading below the optical center), that means giving a round-top bifocal (base-down effect) for balance. For minus lenses, that means giving a flat-top bifocal (Fig. 16.16).

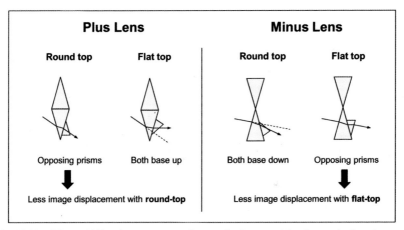

Fig. 16.16 Effect of bifocal segments on image displacement in plus and minus lenses.

For myopic spectacles, flat-top bifocals are best as they minimize both image jump and displacement. For hyperopic spectacles, it is more complicated. Flat-top bifocals minimize image jump but maximize image displacement, while round-top bifocals minimize image displacement but maximize image jump.

In theory, image displacement is probably more of an annoyance than the transient effect of image jump, so round-top bifocals are probably best for patients wearing plus lenses; however, in practice, many opticians give flat-top bifocal segments regardless of the prescription because flat-top segments are less expensive and easier to acquire and assemble. As long as a patient is not complaining, this is acceptable; just remember to consider these issues when you encounter a patient who does not like their new bifocals.

21. **After uneventful bilateral cataract surgery on a famous malpractice lawyer, Ruth Leslie Lawless, you find that her refraction is –4.00 D OD and –1.00 D OS. With a +2 D add, she can read J1+ with each eye. She is orthophoric at distance and does not seem to be bothered by aniseikonia, but she complains of vertical diplopia when reading with her new glasses.**

(a) **The optical centers of the flat-top bifocal segments are 0.5 cm below the optical centers of the distance glasses. Ms. Lawless reads 0.7 cm below the optical centers of her flat-top bifocals. How much prismatic disparity between the eyes is induced in the reading position?**

Net prism 3.6 PD base-down OD (that is, 3.6 PD base-up OS).

If the bifocals are identical (strength and type), the induced vertical prismatic disparity caused by bifocals will cancel out, causing only image displacement (the horizontal prism will not!). In this case, the vertical prism from the bifocal segments does cancel out and may be ignored for the purpose of these calculations. The net induced prism is the difference between the distance correction in the two eyes (Fig. 16.17).

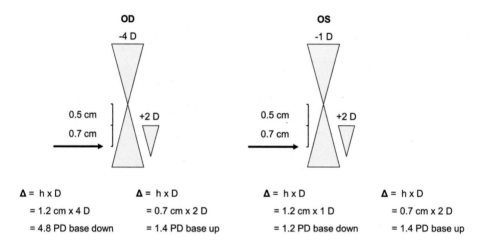

Net Δ = 3.6 PD base down OD or 3.6 PD base up OS

Fig. 16.17 Diagram showing prism effect from glasses and bifocal segments. *OD*, Right eye; *OS*, left eye; *PD*, prism diopters.

(b) **Name some ways to limit the induced prismatic effects of these glasses in the reading position.**

Many patients physiologically adapt or learn to fuse small vertical deviations. While the patient might be able to learn to fuse 3.6 PD of vertical phoria, most people can fuse only 2 to 3 PD of vertical deviation, so there is a good chance she will need to have something done to alleviate her symptoms.

The following methods may help:
- Slab-off prism (bicentric grinding)
- Lower both optical centers to compromise the vertical imbalance between distance and near
- Dissimilar bifocal segments (round-top on one side, flat-top on the other)
- Fresnel prism over one bifocal segment

- Contact lenses instead of glasses
- Separate single vision glasses for distance and near with optical centers properly placed

In practice, many patients do not want to wear contact lenses all day, a Fresnel prism on one bifocal segment is not likely to be tolerated, dissimilar bifocal segments would be cosmetically unacceptable, and lowering the optical centers halfway would still demand a robust vertical fusional amplitude when shifting from distance to near. Slab-off prism is therefore the preferred approach; it can be ground into the more myopic (less hyperopic) lens by any optician. It is not necessary to take all 3.6 PD off—just measure how much is needed in the clinic and specify that amount in the prescription.

22. **You are on call and summoned to the emergency department on a Saturday evening to "clear the globe" of a 9-year-old soccer player prior to urgent repair of an orbital floor fracture by the plastic surgery team. The girl, who wears glasses of plano OD and –3 D OS, presented with double vision after a head butt at a soccer game. The patient confirms that she has diplopia. Cover testing reveals a 6 PD left hypertropia with full extraocular movements. Your review of the CT scan indicates a nondisplaced orbital fracture with no clear evidence of entrapment. The athlete's glasses are bent and crooked.**

   (a) **Assuming there is no muscle entrapment, what is the likely cause of the hypertropia and how can you confirm this?**

   Induced prism from the bent glasses.

   The bent glasses may have displaced the optical center of the left –3 D lens, which is inducing prism. Repeat the measurements with the correction in trial frames to confirm that there is no strabismus.

   (b) **Which direction was the left lens bent to create the impression on cover testing that the left eye is hypertropic?**

   Left lens displaced downward.

   A left hypertropia is created by a base-up prism. For a minus lens, the left lens would need to be displaced downward so that the base-up prism is now in the line of sight.

   (c) **How badly were the glasses bent (in cm) to induce a 6 PD left hypertropia?**

   2 cm downward displacement of –3 D lens.

   There is no power in the right lens, so all the induced prism comes from the displacement of the left lens. Use the equation, $\Delta = h \times P$, and solve for h:

   $$\Delta = h \times P$$
   $$6\,PD = h \times 3\,D$$
   $$h = 2\,cm$$

Therefore the optical center of the -3 D lens was displaced 2 cm downward over the left eye. Fortunately, you are able to pull out your Swiss army knife (which you carry with you at all times), use the needle-nose plier attachment to bend the glasses frames back into shape, and cure the diplopia. Before you head home, you ask the medical student to give the plastic surgery fellow the great news that you have "cleared the globe," and not only that, the orbits are fine and you have canceled the procedure.

CHAPTER 17

Instruments

1. What principle is the manual lensmeter based on? How does it work?

The optometer (Badal) principle.

An illuminated mobile target is moved back and forth along the optical axis of an unknown lens until the vergence leaving the lens is zero. The target is viewed with a telescope that provides magnification and reduces the effect of the observer's accommodation and refractive error, allowing precise detection of parallel rays at neutralization. Without the addition of a second lens, called a fixed (or "optometer") lens, a lensmeter would have a very nonlinear dial. That is, the dial would have to be turned a large amount when going from 1 to 2 diopters (D) and a microscopic amount when going from 14 to 15 D. The fixed lens is carefully positioned so that its focal plane exactly coincides with the location of the unknown lens (Fig. 17.1). The observer moves the illuminated mobile target back and forth behind the fixed lens; this varies the vergence entering the fixed lens. The linear distance of the target from the rear focal plane of the fixed lens is then directly proportional to the power of the unknown lens.

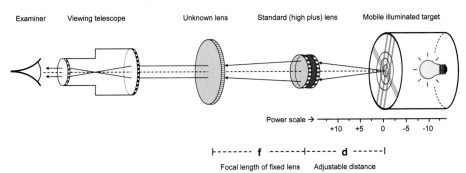

Fig. 17.1 Optometer (Badal) principle that underlies the manual lensmeter.

2. How does one measure prism power and decentration of the optical centers in glasses?

With a lensmeter.

Have the patient fixate on your eye and mark the glasses with a felt marker where the line of sight intersects the lenses. Place the glasses in the lensmeter with the mark centered in the nose cone of the lensmeter. If the lensmeter cross target is not centered, prismatic power is present. This power may be due *either* to ground-in prism or to decentration. If you cannot find a position where the cross target is centered, then some of the prism is ground in. If you can find a position where the cross target is centered, some of the prism is due to decentration, but there may also be some ground-in prismatic power, especially in high-power lenses. This is why it is important to mark the intersection of the line of sight with the lenses to measure effective prism power (as experienced by the patient) accurately.

The amount of prismatic power may be read off the scale in the lensmeter eyepiece. If the lensmeter cross target is deflected *down* to the circle marked "1," then there is 1 prism diopter (PD) of base-*down* prism. If the cross target is off the scale, you must use a handheld prism with its base oriented in the direction opposite the prismatic power to determine the amount of power. For example, if the cross target is centered when a 10 PD prism is placed base *up* in the lensmeter light path, the glasses must have 10 PD of base-*down* prism (some lensmeter designs include an adjustable prism that allows you to dial in a neutralizing power instead of having to use a handheld prism).

3. What optics principle is the foundation of most autorefractors?

The Scheiner principle.

This principle is based on the fact that if a distant light is viewed through a double-pinhole aperture, a person with emmetropia will see a single light while a person with ametropia (hyperopic or myopic) will see two lights (Fig. 17.2). A form of this principle is used in most autorefractors.

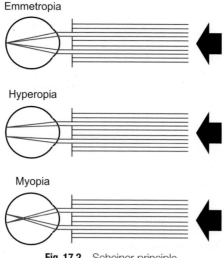

Fig. 17.2 Scheiner principle.

4. What are the origins of "with" and "against" motion during retinoscopy?

At neutralization, the far point of the eye coincides with the peephole of the retinoscope, and all the light returning from the eye passes through the peephole to the examiner. Thus the pupil seems to fill with light (Fig. 17.3, *left*).

When the far point of the eye is in front of or behind the examiner, only part of the light returning from the eye passes through the peephole. Thus the pupil is bright where the originating light rays pass through the peephole, and dark where the returning light is blocked, creating the appearance of a streak.

If the patient's eye has too much plus power (far point between the observer and the patient), the light rays cross at the far point and are inverted before they reach the examiner. This causes the streak to appear to move opposite to the illumination and "against" motion is seen (Fig. 17.3, *right*). If not enough plus power is present (far point beyond the peephole), the light rays have not yet crossed at the far point before entering the retinoscope. Therefore they are not inverted and "with" motion is observed (Fig. 17.3, *middle*).

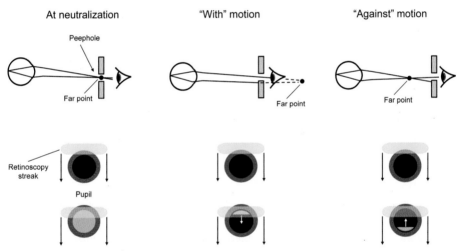

Fig. 17.3 Retinoscopy reflex. At neutrality *(left)*, when the far point is behind the eye *(middle)*, and when the far point is in front of the eye *(right)*.

5. What is optical doubling, why is it useful, and what instruments use it?

Optical doubling (or image doubling) is used to measure small distances in a moving patient with great precision. Theoretically, you could simply engrave a reticle (scale) on an eyepiece and measure the object of interest (e.g., the width of a magnified image of a corneal cross-section) (Fig. 17.4, *left*). However, this is not practical, since a patient must remain virtually motionless while the reticle is lined up with the magnified image. Instead, imagine that the field of view can be split into upper and lower halves. Now imagine that the lower half is shifted to the right with a prism (Fig. 17.4, *right*). The prism power can be adjusted until the left side of the lower image (corneal epithelium in this example) lines up with the right side of the upper image (corneal endothelium). With a doubling prism, the separation of the two images does not change when the patient moves (since both images move together). The actual size (thickness in this example) of the image can be calculated from the power of the prism required to align the images.

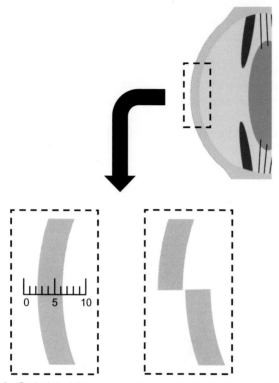

Fig. 17.4 Optical doubling; removes the need to try to align a stationary ruler with a moving target.

Optical doubling is used in keratometry (for both Bausch & Lomb keratometers, which use constant mire size and variable image doubling, and Javal-Schiotz keratometers, which use constant image doubling with adjustable mire separation), pachymetry, and applanation tonometry.

6. What does a manual keratometer *actually* measure? How does it convert this value into a keratometry measurement?

A manual keratometer measures the size of an image that is reflected by the cornea. The size is measured precisely using optical doubling (see Question 5 above). The object (mire) is of a known size, and the ratio of object to image size is used to calculate the magnifying power of a small (3-mm) annulus of the cornea. The magnification is in turn used to calculate the radius of curvature (in mm) of the cornea using the formula for the power of a mirror, $P = -2/r$ (see Chapter 3, Mirrors).

This gives us the radius of curvature of the cornea, which we can use to estimate the *refractive* power (the keratometer directly measures the *reflective* power, which is not the same as refractive power). Since we know the radius of curvature, we can infer the refractive power using the formula:

$$P = \frac{(n'-n)}{r} = \frac{(1.3375-1)}{r} = \frac{0.3375}{r}$$

n′ = keratometric refractive index = 1.3375
n = index of refraction of air = 1.000
r = radius of curvature in meters (measured by keratometer)

This translates the radius of curvature (measured by the manual keratometer) to a refractive power in diopters. Why do we need a "keratometric refractive index" (n = 1.3375) instead of using the actual refractive index of the cornea (n = 1.376)? Because the posterior surface of the cornea acts as a minus lens. The posterior corneal curvature is not measured by a manual keratometer, so the refractive index needs to be adjusted (1.376 → 1.3375) to account for the contribution of the posterior cornea. More advanced techniques, such as corneal tomography, can directly measure the posterior corneal surface.

7. How does automated keratometry work?

Some automated keratometers work by projecting several pairs of lights onto the cornea (on opposite sides of the line of sight) and measuring the distance between the reflected lights (e.g., IOLMaster keratometer). A steeper meridian will cause the lights to be closer together while a flatter meridian will cause the lights to be farther apart. The distance between the points is used to calculate the anterior corneal curvature, which is then converted into an estimated refractive power. Automated keratometry can also be performed with corneal topography or corneal tomography (see Question 8 below).

8. Are there modalities to evaluate the anterior corneal surface in detail? What about the posterior corneal surface? How do they work?

There are widely used modalities able to perform *corneal topography* (characterizing the anterior corneal surface) and *corneal tomography* (generating a 3D recreation of the cornea to measure both the anterior and posterior corneal surfaces and corneal thickness). It is useful to be aware of the underlying optical principles of commonly used techniques.

1. *Placido disk:* This technique uses concentric rings reflected by the anterior corneal surface. The distance between the reflected rings and the regularity (or irregularity) of the reflected rings can be assessed subjectively, or a computerized quantitative assessment of the entire anterior corneal surface can be generated (e.g., Atlas, OPD-Scan).
2. *Scanning slit:* Rapidly scanning slit beams of light are projected onto the cornea and a camera captures the reflected beams to create a map of the anterior and posterior corneal surfaces (e.g., OrbScan).
3. *Scheimpflug imaging:* This uses a monochromatic slit light source with a camera that rotates around the optical axis of the eye (e.g., PentaCam). This method corrects for the nonplanar shape of the cornea to improve accuracy.

9. What basic principle was revolutionary in the development of the slit lamp?

A *common pivot point*.

A slit lamp has an illumination system and a viewing system; the illuminated slit is imaged precisely over the common pivot point of the illumination and viewing paths. This allows both the slit beam and the object of regard to remain in precise focus at all times.

10. How does an applanation tonometer work? What do the numbers on the scale mean? Can errors be induced when measuring an astigmatic cornea? What if a patient has had refractive surgery for high myopia?

In an applanation tonometer, increasing force is placed against the cornea to flatten (applanate) its curved surface. When the applanated area is exactly 3.06 mm in diameter (not area!), the force against the eye in dynes times 10 yields the intraocular pressure (IOP) in mm Hg. The numbers on the scale are the dynes of force pressed against the eye, which is why you need to multiple by 10 to get the IOP. To increase the accuracy of identifying the point where 3.06 mm of corneal diameter has been applanated, a split-field plastic prism in the tonometer tip separates the half fields by 3.06 mm (i.e., optical doubling). The measurement is completed when the inner edges of the tear meniscus semicircles are aligned.

If significant corneal astigmatism is present, the applanated area will be an ellipse rather than a circle. You can compensate by rotating the prism to *align the red mark* with the axis of the *minus cylinder* correction. Another accurate way to avoid error in astigmatic corneas is to applanate twice: once with the split prism horizontal and once with it vertical. The true pressure is the average of the two readings. Astigmatic errors become measurable with more than 4 D of corneal cylinder, but even 4 D of corneal cylinder causes an error of only 1 mm Hg.

The accuracy of applanation tonometry depends on assumptions that the corneal rigidity and thickness are relatively constant among individuals. A thinner cornea (e.g., post-LASIK) may cause an underestimation of the true intraocular pressure. For this reason, patients with thinner corneas are considered to be at higher risk for glaucoma, and some ophthalmologists use corneal pachymetry values (see Question 11 below) to calcluate a corrected IOP.

11. What does a pachymeter measure? What are the methods of performing pachymetry?

Pachymetry measures the corneal thickness.

There are several methods, including ultrasound (sound waves), specular microscopy (reflections of light from the anterior and posterior corneal surface), and optical coherence tomography (interference pattern of reflected laser light).

12. How does a specular microscope work? What is being "counted"?

By using reflection from the interface between the endothelial cells and the aqueous humor, the endothelial cells can be visualized and counted. The illumination path and viewing path must be separated so the bright reflections from the anterior corneal surface do not obscure the endothelium.

13. Discuss the principles of fluorescein angiography.

Sodium fluorescein dye is injected into a vein where 60–80% is bound to serum albumin and 20–40% remains unbound. Fluorescein has a maximum absorption at 485 nm and peak fluorescence at 530 nm. A white flash from the camera passes through an interference filter, and blue light enters the eye. The fluorescein absorbs the blue light and emits longer-wavelength yellow-green (530 nm) light, along with the reflected blue light. A blue-blocking interference filter is placed in front of the camera to prevent the reflected blue wavelengths from entering the camera. The light emitted in the yellow-green wavelengths is imaged onto a detector optimized for high-contrast imaging.

14. How is indocyanine green (ICG) angiography different from fluorescein angiography?

In fluorescein angiography, the largest portion of light energy during excitation and emission is absorbed by the retinal pigment epithelium (RPE) and macular xanthophyll, which can make it difficult to visualize certain choroidal vascular patterns. Furthermore, unbound fluorescein leaks rapidly from the highly fenestrated choriocapillaris.

In contrast, ICG is highly (98%) bound to plasma proteins. ICG has a maximum absorption and peak fluorescence at 805 nm and 835 nm, respectively. Because this falls in the near-infrared part of the spectrum, the light more readily penetrates the RPE and macular xanthophyll, and the choroidal circulation is more easily visualized.

15. How does OCT work? Why is an OCT image so much more detailed than an ultrasound image?

In OCT, coherent, directional light is bounced off an ocular structure such as the retina. As the light waves pass through tissue, they are slowed in different amounts depending on the composition of the tissue. To detect the changes, a second coherent beam of light is split off of the first and bounced off of a mirror that is the same distance from the source as the tissue (the "reference arm"). The varying phase and/or frequency of the two light beams creates interference, which is detected by combining the waves in an interferometer. The variations are computed to create an "A scan"-type image. As with ultrasound, a series of A scans are then combined to create a two-dimensional B scan image. Because light has a much higher frequency (shorter wavelength) than sound, OCT images have much higher resolution than ultrasound images.

16. For a mass in the ciliary body, would you prefer an anterior segment OCT (AS-OCT) or ultrasound biomicroscopy (UBM)? Why?

UBM is preferable.

Both AS-OCT and UBM can be used to image the anterior segment in detail. AS-OCT uses interference patterns from reflected light while UBM uses sound waves. While AS-OCT is easier for patients, light waves from an OCT device cannot penetrate the iris. In contrast, sound waves (including ultrasound waves) pass through the iris, so UBM is generally better able to characterize lesions in the ciliary body.

17. **What is the angular magnification of a 20 D lens when used as a simple magnifier?**

    5× angular magnification (at 25 cm).

    A simple magnifier is a plus lens used to increase the angular subtense of a near object. The magnifying power is always expressed relative to an arbitrary reference distance. A conventional reference distance of 25 cm was established long ago. The formula for angular magnification is equal to the dioptric power of the lens divided by 4:

    > Simple magnifier, angular magnification = P/4

    Thus a 20 D condensing lens has a magnification of (20/4) = 5× (relative to a reference distance of 25 cm) when used as a simple magnifier.

18. **What is the angular magnification of a 20 D lens when used as a simple magnifier if the reference distance is changed to 40 cm?**

    8× angular magnification (at 40 cm).

    For the conventional reference distance of 25 cm, Mag = P/4 or Mag = P ∗ 0.25 m. If you remember the formula as Mag = D ∗ reference distance (in m), then you can calculate the angular magnification of a simple magnifier for any reference distance. For a 40-cm reference distance, Mag = D ∗ 0.40 m = 20 ∗ 0.40 m = 8× That is, an object viewed through a 20 D lens used as a simple magnifier takes up eight times more of your visual field than it would if it were held 40 cm away and viewed without magnification.

19. **What is the magnification of the retina of a person with emmetropia when viewed with a direct ophthalmoscope? What type of magnification is this?**

    15× angular magnification (assuming normal eye power of 60 D).

    The direct ophthalmoscope uses the patient's eye as a simple magnifier. Since the formula for a simple magnifier is Mag = D/4 and the power of the normal eye is 60 D, the magnification is 60/4 = 15×. This is angular magnification, and relative to a reference distance of 25 cm (i.e., the retina appears to be 15× larger than if you cut the eye in half and looked at the retina without magnification from a distance of 25 cm).

20. **A first-year medical student in Physical Diagnosis class is assigned to examine the optic disk of his clinical skills partner using a direct ophthalmoscope. By some miracle, he is able to see the disk. While celebrating success and taking another look, he knocks the partner's contact lens out of her eye. The lens cannot be found, but he is so enchanted by the view that he begs to take one more look, this time without the contact lens in place. After a 20-minute effort, he again**

manages to view the partner's optic disk, but this time it seems to be much larger. Why?

The partner likely has high myopia.

In patients with myopia, the eye has more built-in plus power than it needs (in optics vernacular, it contains a plus error lens). When the contact lens was dislodged, the medical student had to dial minus power into the ophthalmoscope to once again see the retina clearly. This minus lens forms the eyepiece of a Galilean telescope. The student was therefore looking at his partner's fundus through a Galilean telescope, providing him with a magnified image of the partner's optic disk. The increased magnification also reduces the field of view, making the medical student's accomplishment of finding the optic disk after the contact lens had been dislodged all the more remarkable. If the partner had hyperopia, the opposite would have occurred: the disk would have looked smaller (and the field of view would have been somewhat larger, making the disk easier to find).

21. **What is axial magnification? If you change the transverse magnification of an optical system, what happens to the axial magnification? What are the consequences?**

Axial magnification is *magnification along the optical axis (depth)*. It is equal to the square of the transverse magnification:

$$(\text{Mag}_{\text{axial}}) = (\text{Mag}_{\text{transverse}})^2$$

Therefore if you increase the transverse magnification, there is an even greater increase in the axial magnification. The consequences are that the magnified image is distorted: there is a greater increase in the appearance of depth relative to the appearance of the height/width (Fig. 17.5).

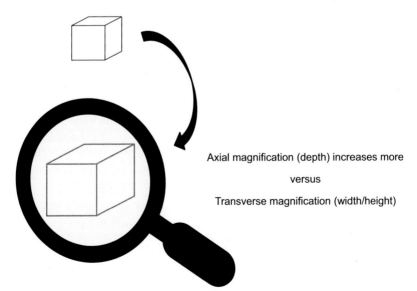

Axial magnification (depth) increases more

versus

Transverse magnification (width/height)

Fig. 17.5 Diagram showing the relative effect of axial versus transverse magnification.

22. Describe how a binocular indirect ophthalmoscope works.

The binocular indirect ophthalmoscope has an illumination source and a viewing system. Both the illumination and viewing paths pass through the handheld condensing lens. A mirror places the light source closer to the examiner's eyes. The binocular eyepieces contain reflective surfaces to reduce the observer's interpupillary distance to about 15 mm. This allows both examiner's eyes, along with the illumination source, to be imaged within the patient's dilated pupil, giving the examiner a well-lit and *binocular* view. A real, inverted image of the patient's retina is formed between the condensing lens and the observer. This aerial image is viewed by the examiner (Fig. 17.6).

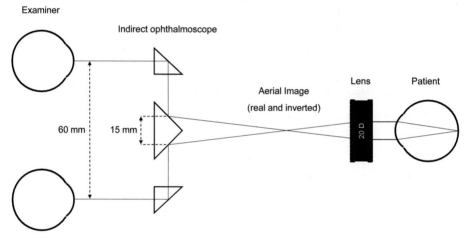

Fig. 17.6 Schematic of an indirect ophthalmoscope. The eyepieces reduce interpupillary distance from 60 mm to 15 mm. The examiner views a real, inverted image which is formed between the lens and observer.

23. How does the small-pupil setting on an indirect ophthalmoscope work? What is the tradeoff?

The small-pupil setting decreases the interpupillary distance even further (and may move the light source closer to the eyes as well). This allows both eyes and the light source to be imaged through a smaller pupil. The trade-off is decreased depth perception and increased glare from reflections. Since most indirect ophthalmoscopes now offer a small-pupil setting, you should routinely check to see that the small-pupil setting is not selected before use so that you do not compromise the quality of your view in a well-dilated patient.

24. What is the magnification (transverse and axial) of the image of the retina of a patient with emmetropia using a 20 D condensing lens?

Transverse magnification 3×; Axial magnification (perceived) 2.25×.

The transverse magnification of the aerial image of the retina of a patient with emmetropia is the ratio of the power of the patient's eye (60 D) to the power of the condensing lens. Thus for a 20 D condensing lens, the transverse magnification is $60/20 = 3\times$. The axial magnification—how deep or high a fundus lesion looks—is the square of the transverse magnification $\rightarrow 3^2 = 9\times$. However, our interpupillary distance is reduced from 60 to 15 mm (see Fig. 17.6), reducing our stereoscopic clues fourfold, and this reduces the *perceived* axial magnification of a 20 D condensing lens to $9/4 = 2.25\times$. Overall, you get a magnified view that is slightly flattened; that is, some degree of depth distortion.

25. Which lens gives the least distortion of depth during indirect ophthalmoscopy: a 15 D, 20 D, or 30 D indirect ophthalmoscope lens? Why?

A 15 D lens gives the least distortion of depth.

Use the calculations like those in Question 24 (Table 17.1). This does not mean that you should throw away your 20 D lens in exchange for a 15 D lens. It is just a caution that the appearance of depth will change depending on which condensing lens is used.

TABLE 17.1 ■ **Magnification and Depth Distortion When Using Different Indirect Ophthalmoscopy Lenses**

P	$Mag_{trans} =$ 60 D/lens power	$Mag_{ax} =$ Mag_{trans}^2	Perceived $Mag_{ax} =$ $Mag_{ax}/4$	Depth Distortion = Perceived Mag_{ax}/Mag_{trans}
30 D	2×	4×	1×	0.50
20 D	3×	9×	2.25×	0.75
15 D	4×	16×	4×	1.00

P, lens power; *Mag_{trans}*, transverse magnification; *Mag_{ax}*, axial magnification

26. You and a rescued space explorer, Major Tom, are stranded on a lost planet with your trial lens set, but only a few lenses survived the crash landing. You are left with a –20.00 D sphere, +4.00 D sphere, +5.00 D sphere, and +20.00 D sphere. You build a viewing device to search the stars for rescue craft using the –20.00 and +4.00 lenses. Major Tom uses the +20.00 and +5.00 lenses. Major Tom complains that his telescope seems to be inferior to yours.

(a) **What did each of you build?**

You built a Galilean telescope (using the –20 D lens as the eyepiece and the +4 D lens as the objective). Major Tom built an astronomical telescope (using the +20 D as the eyepiece and the +5 D lens as the objective).

(b) **How far apart are the lenses for each telescope?**

Galilean telescope: 20 cm; astronomical telescope: 25 cm.

For the Galilean telescope, the length is the difference between the focal lengths of the lenses. The difference between 25 cm (4 D lens) and 5 cm (20 D lens) is 20 cm. For the astronomical telescope, the length is the *sum* of the focal lengths. So, 20 cm (5 D lens) + 5 cm (20 D lens) = 25 cm.

(c) Which telescope will provide you with more magnification?

Galilean (5×) > Astronomical (4×).

The angular magnification of a telescope is equal to the power of the eyepiece divided by the power of the objective. The magnification of the Galilean telescope is 20/4 = 5×, and the magnification of the astronomical telescope is 20/5 = 4×.

(d) Will the telescopes have upright or inverted images?

Galilean: upright; astronomical: inverted

The Galilean telescope will provide an upright image of approaching ships, while Major Tom's astronomical telescope will produce an inverted image.

For all of these reasons, you chose the superior telescope.

EXAM PEARL

A high-yield exam topic is the difference between Galilean and astronomical (or Keplerian) telescopes (Table 17.2).

TABLE 17.2 ■ Key Differences Between Astronomical and Galilean Telescopes

Type of Telescope	Astronomical	Galilean
Eyepiece	Plus	Minus
Objective	Plus	Plus
Distance between lenses	Sum of focal lengths	Difference in focal length
Image orientation	Inverted	Upright
Angular magnification	$Mag_{Angular} = -\dfrac{P_{eyepiece}}{P_{objective}}$	$Mag_{Angular} = -\dfrac{P_{eyepiece}}{P_{objective}}$

---

27. How is a Galilean telescope modified when used as a surgical loupe?

The binocular surgical loupe is just a short Galilean telescope fitted with an add to bring the working distance from infinity up to the preferred working distance. To calculate the power of the add for any loupes, take the reciprocal of the working distance in meters.

28. A telescope is made using a +25 D objective and –50 D eyepiece. Another telescope is made using a +5 D objective and –10 D eyepiece. Which telescope has greater angular magnification? Which would be a better choice for surgical loupes?

Both have angular magnification of 2×. The first telescope is much shorter (2 cm vs 10 cm) and therefore a better choice for Loupes.

The angular magnification is equal to -Peyepiece/Pobjective, which is equal to 2× for both telescopes. The length of a Galilean telescope is the difference between the focal lengths of the lenses. For the +25 D lens (f = 4 cm) and the −50 D lens (f = 2 cm), the length is 4–2 = 2 cm. For the +5 D lens (f = 20 cm) and the −10 D lens (f = 10 cm), the length is 20–10 = 10 cm. This is why powerful lenses are used to make surgical loupes.

CHAPTER 18

Low Vision

1. When should low-vision aids be offered?

Low-vision aids should be offered when a patient's visual needs exceed his or her visual capabilities. This may occur with a visual acuity of 20/40 in one patient and 20/200 in another.

2. Describe the steps you would take in the evaluation of a 52-year-old man with low vision.

History:
- Duration and course of visual loss (may influence his motivation and acceptance of aids)
- Current occupational and avocational needs
- Other physical limitations (e.g., tremor, deafness)
- Prior use of visual aids
- Comfort with use of technology
- Expectations and acceptance of available aids

Examination:
- Full eye examination to assess the cause of vision loss
- Precise refraction, with distance and near visual acuity (move patient closer if unable to see largest letter on chart)
- Other findings that may influence the type of aid prescribed should be noted (e.g., nystagmus, photophobia, aniridia, or visual field defects)

Trial of a variety of low-vision aids:
- Trial of aids that seem appropriate to needs and capabilities
- Many patients need more than one low-vision aid

Depending on the patient's stamina, it may take more than one visit to complete this encounter.

3. A patient has low vision and manifest latent nystagmus. How should you measure visual acuity?

If a patient has nystagmus with a latent component, monocular occlusion will exaggerate the nystagmus, which will reduce measured visual acuity. In such cases, fog the fellow eye with a high plus lens rather than covering it with an occluder. Measure visual acuity under binocular conditions as well. Nystagmus patients with a null point should also be allowed to adopt a compensatory head posture for best visual acuity.

4. You are seeing 80-year-old twins. Both have low vision, one due to macular degeneration and the other due to advanced glaucoma. Would you recommend the same low-vision aids?

Probably not. Twin 1 likely has central vision loss from macular degeneration while twin 2 likely has peripheral vision loss from glaucoma. These two types of vision loss require different approaches.

Patients with *central vision loss* usually need *magnification*. You can increase the size of objects (e.g., large text) or use optical devices such as high-power adds, stand/hand magnifiers, or loupes.

Patients with *peripheral vision loss* usually need help with *orientation and mobility* (magnification could make a small visual field worse). This can be achieved with a cane, seeing-eye dog, or environmental modifications. Optical methods of addressing peripheral vision loss (minification, partial prism) are in development but not widely utilized.

5. Discuss nonoptical modalities in the treatment of low vision.

When encountering a patient with low-vision needs, it can be tempting to jump right to the technical details of various optical aids. Do not forget about *nonoptical aids*, which are effective and often easier to implement. These include templates, magic markers, signature guides, high-contrast materials, and good lighting as well as large-print books, playing cards, telephones, watches, and timers. The wide availability of smartphones and other computer technology has made access to nonoptical aids such as tablets, screen readers, and magnifying applications much more accessible. Absorptive lenses can help people who are bothered by glare (such as patients with aniridia and albinism) or who see better in lower light levels (patients with congenital achromatopsia do best with a very dark *red* lens).

6. A 70-year-old man has a best-corrected visual acuity of 20/100 in each eye and when measured binocularly. He has measurable stereopsis.

(a) What power add should allow him to read newspaper print? Could there be an issue with binocularity? Why and how do you help?

+5 diopter (D) add; may also need 7 prism diopter (PD) base-in prism in both eyes to help maintain binocularity.

Kestenbaum's rule can help you estimate the strength of a near add (or single vision spectacles) that will allow a low-vision patient to read newspaper print (M1, J5, 8 point).

$$\text{Kestenbaum's rule: power of add} = \frac{1}{Va} - AA$$

Va is the visual acuity (Snellen or Early Treatment of Diabetic Retinopathy Study chart).

AA is the amount of accommodation the patient can use comfortably. (You can assume 1/2 of the accommodative amplitude unless otherwise specified.)

Subtraction of the AA is generally not used for older adults.

For our 70-year-old patient with

$$20/100 \text{ visual acuity}, P = 1/Va = 1/(20/100) = 5 \text{ D}$$

With a +5 D add, the patient will need to read at 20 cm – very close to his face. With the materials that close, he may not be able to converge sufficiently to maintain fusion. Therefore you may need to give base-in prism in both eyes. A handy rule of thumb is to give 2 PD more than the power, so in this case you would add 7 PD base-in prism in both eyes (this works for add powers of 4–12 D). The 5 D add and the 7 PD base-in prism for the eye should serve as a starting point. You must still put the lenses in trial frames to test the power and see whether the patient can tolerate the add.

(b) What if this was an 8-year-old child with optic atrophy and 20/100 vision?

Likely no need for an add.

An 8-year-old child should have plenty of accommodation to hold things close to read (remember the AA in the equation). Therefore no add is needed. Her accommodative abilities can be assessed by allowing her to hold the near card as close as she likes while you check near visual acuity and perform dynamic retinoscopy. Not that any 8-year-old child would ever read a newspaper. (What is a "newspaper," anyway?)

7. What are the advantages and disadvantages of a high power add?

Advantages: large field of view, hands-free, easy to use, portable.

Disadvantages: short working distance, heavy.

8. What are the similarities between stand magnifiers and hand magnifiers? What are the relative advantages of each?

Both are aids for near, have variable eye-to-magnifier distance, and can be used with or without a reading add.

Hand magnifiers are inexpensive, easily obtained, and easy to carry. However, they have a small field of view when held farther from the eye and may be difficult to use for patients who have issues with dexterity (e.g., stroke, tremor, or arthritis).

Stand magnifiers are easier for patients with stroke, tremor, or arthritis, but are bulkier and harder to carry in a pocket or purse. Stand magnifiers come with fixed distance or with adjustable height.

9. Dr. Rudy Canal is a 57-year-old dentist who has early-onset macular degeneration and a best-corrected visual acuity of 20/50. He loves his job and would like to keep working as long as possible. Should you prescribe a hand magnifier? If not, are there other options?

A hand magnifier is clearly inappropriate, as dentists need both hands free for their work. Higher-power adds with base-in prism might be considered, but only momentarily, as dentists might prefer not to have a 5-cm working distance while operating a whirling, whining drill deep inside of patients' mouths.

Surgical loupes would likely be the best bet, as Dr. Canal could get higher magnification with a reasonable working distance. Surgical loupes are not for everyone, as they are expensive, have a limited depth of focus, and are conspicuous. But they do allow hands-free magnification with a long working distance and are the best option in this situation.

10. When is a telescope useful for a patient with low vision?

A *telescope* is used when a patient needs better visual acuity *at distance* than can be achieved with spectacle correction alone. Telescopes can be spectacle-mounted (binocular or monocular) or handheld. Patients typically use them to see smaller objects at a distance, such as bus signs or street signs. Spectacle-mounted telescopes are cosmetically obvious and heavy, and all telescopes have a limited field of view.

EXAM PEARL

Remember that all optical aids are used for near vision except for the *telescope*, the only optical aid for *distance*. There are nonoptical aids that are useful for distance, including aids for mobility and orientation and electronic aids to assist with object identification. (A telescope could be used for near with the addition of a plus lens; this is how loupes work.)

11. Mr. Izzy Real has low vision and reports seeing vivid patterns that other people do not see. Has he developed a superpower?

Probably not. Up to one-third of visually impaired persons experience hallucinations. This phenomenon, which is called *Charles Bonnet Syndrome*, can be diagnosed if there are four characteristics present:

1. Preexisting vision loss
2. Vivid, recurrent visual hallucinations
3. Insight into the unreality when it is explained
4. No neurologic or psychiatric disease that could explain hallucinations

Patients will often be reluctant to disclose hallucinations. The main treatment is reassurance. Patients are often relieved to learn what they are seeing and that it is not a sign of underlying psychiatric disease. Antipsychotics are not indicated, but discontinuation of proton pump inhibitors (if used) may be helpful. (If Mr. Real *has* developed a superpower, then you should help him design a snazzy logo and offer your services as a master of optics and lasers, working silently and tirelessly in the background to help him fight for truth, justice, and a better tomorrow.)

CHAPTER 19

Good People, Bad Optics: The Dissatisfied Patient

Being an ophthalmologist is the best job in the world. Seriously, it is amazing, especially pediatric ophthalmology (really!). But you will have to deal with challenging patients (on exams *and* in real life). Many of the issues that cause patient dissatisfaction are either related to optics or can be solved using optics. Here are some common scenarios with an optics slant that may help you keep your patients (and your examiners) happy, even if you are not having the best day yourself.

1. **Your first patient of the day, Noah Copay, is here for an "urgent" follow-up visit and immediately notes that you arrived at the clinic 32 seconds after his appointment was scheduled. He just spent $1200 on his first new pair of glasses in 15 years. He now reports that "your prescription makes my eyes feel like they are being sucked out of my head." What should you do?**

   This is one of many colorful ways that patients use to describe their response to subtle but unfavorable changes in lens design or positioning. Check the location of optical centers for induced prism, check bifocal segment height (including progressive bifocals) and frame alignment, compare the base curve of the new lenses to that of his old lenses, and look for cylinder that has been ground into the front (very rare) versus the back of the lens. The last two items require the use of a lens clock.

2. **Your next patient, Dr. Colin M. Dee, is a family practitioner who happens to be your best referral source, and whom you refracted as a favor. You even took extra time to put the refraction in trial frames to make sure he was happy with the refraction before writing out the prescription. He is returning with his new glasses, complaining (very nicely) that his vision just does not seem to be as sharp as it was in your office at the end of the last refraction. What are some possible causes?**

   Check that the prescription was filled correctly. Is there an uncompensated change in vertex distance? The pantoscopic tilt, base curve, and aperture size of trial lenses placed in trial frames are likely to be different than with prescribed glasses, so there may be some aspect of how they were made that is not comfortable, especially in combination with a large change in prescription (particularly a change in cylinder). Consider putting the exact same prescription in trial frames again to see if it is still satisfactory. Of course, you may have refracted him incorrectly (check pinhole acuity with the new glasses) or you may need to adjust the prescription for infinity to compensate for the 20-foot eye lane.

3. **Your next patient, Ms. Presby, has early cataracts, but at the last visit you were able to correct her to 20/15 in each eye with a change in prescription. She hands you the new bifocals (with her pinky finger extended), complaining, "I can't read with the new pair you gave me, doctor." Her old prescription is +1.50 –1.50 × 90 in both eyes (OU), also with a +1.50 add. Her new pair is +0.75 −2.00 × 90 OU, with a +1.50 add. Distance visual acuity is still 20/15 with the new lenses, and lower with the old lenses. What happened?**

Loss of plus power at near.

When you change the spherical equivalent of glasses, you should adjust the add to keep the same power for reading. The near power through a bifocal is equal to the spherical equivalent of the distance portion of the glasses plus the reading add. In the old glasses, the total power at near was +2.25 OU (+0.75 spherical equivalent plus +1.50 add), while the new glasses have a total near power of +1.25 OU (–0.25 plus +1.50). Since you decreased the spherical equivalent by +1.00 in the distance portion of the glasses, you need to add +1.00 to the reading add and give a +2.50 add to maintain the same total power for near.

4. **You hear screaming in the next room. After a deep breath, you go past the billing office (where the screaming is coming from) and enter the exam room to find Hugh G. Monster Jr., an 18-month-old boy with high hyperopia, fully accommodative esotropia (orthotropic with glasses), and mild left amblyopia. His parents say that absolutely refuses to wear the glasses you prescribed. What might you suggest?**

Make sure his parents understand how important the glasses are to the development and maintenance of their son's visual development and eye alignment. Parents often have trouble believing their perfect child could possibly need glasses, especially when the child seems to see just fine. Second, make sure the glasses actually fit. Opticians often fit small children and infants with frames that are too big for their faces. Be sure to suggest an optician who has an interest and expertise in fitting children's glasses. Also consider that children are tough on glasses, and parents should expect to have the frames adjusted frequently. If the earpiece is digging into the ear of an adult, he or she will complain about it, but a child will just drop the glasses in the toilet or bury them in the sandbox. Finally, it may be worth rechecking the cycloplegic refraction to ensure that the prescription is correct.

If a child with hyperopia will not wear glasses despite encouragement, consider a short course of cycloplegia to paralyze accommodation and make the child more appreciative of the improvement in visual acuity. Sometimes it is necessary to put the efforts on hold for a few weeks or months and try again.

5. **Just before lunch, you see Lon Gise, a 32-year-old man with high myopia. At the last appointment, he asked for glasses with thinner lenses, so, having studied *Last-Minute Optics* the night before to help you fall asleep, you recommended high-index lenses. Lon returns saying that he cannot see as well with the new glasses. Corrected visual acuity is 20/15 in each eye. What might be the reason?**

Although high-index lenses are thinner and lighter than conventional plastic lenses, they can have more chromatic aberration (low Abbe number), especially in higher powers, depending on the exact lens material used. When a white spot is viewed away from the optical center, it will have a blue or yellow "ghost" or shadow (prismatic effect). Also, the "sweet spot," the area of the lens giving the clearest vision, can be smaller with high-index lenses. The optician should be able to find the right compromise among lens thickness, sweet spot, and Abbe number to address the patient's concerns.

6. **You must skip lunch because of an urgent visit with a 56-year-old man, Kal Aheed, who presented to the emergency department of the local hospital with a 1-week history of diplopia. He recieved a CAT scan, a PET scan, an MRI, and an MRA. All were negative. Then his vet ordered a PET scan for his cat. Someone suggested it might be a good idea to see an eye doctor.**

   (a) **What key ocular historical points do you need to elicit in a patient with new-onset double vision?**

   ■ Is the diplopia still present with one eye closed (differentiate monocular vs. binocular diplopia)?
   ■ How sudden was the onset?
   ■ Any prior history of diplopia?
   ■ Does it change throughout the day (variable strabismus might suggest myasthenia gravis)?
   ■ Are the images separated vertically, horizontally, or both?
   ■ Is one image tilted? (It can be difficult to separate oblique diplopia from torsional diplopia.)

   (b) **During cover testing, he reports that the double vision disappears when the left eye is covered but remains when the right eye is covered. What is this called and how would you assess it?**

   Monocular diplopia of the left eye.

   Monocular diplopia is usually caused by irregularities in the refractive surfaces of the eyes (e.g., dry eye, corneal epithelial irregularities, stromal scarring, refractive surgery, uncorrected refractive error, or incipient cataract). Nonoptical causes such as retinal irregularities are extremely rare. The key diagnostic step is to see whether the diplopia improves through a pinhole occluder, as optically induced monocular diplopia is almost always reduced or eliminated by the pinhole. If it remains with the pinhole occluder in place, then the problem could be with the retina, or it may be functional vision loss (also known as factitious, nonorganic, or nonphysiologic vision loss). Correction of refractive error and/or treatment of dry eye is often enough to reduce or eliminate the problem.

7. **Your first afternoon patient, Dee Plopia, is a 46-year-old woman who also presents with double vision. You say to yourself, "I'm a comprehensive ophthalmologist, I**

didn't sign up for adult strabismus, pediatric ophthalmology, or neuro-ophthalmology. Doesn't anybody need cataract surgery today?" In this case, Dee thinks that the problem occurred either just before or just after you changed her glasses prescription 6 months ago, but then again, maybe she has had double vision for years. The double vision is binocular. Cover testing with correction reveals a right hypertropia of 4 prism diopters (PD), worse in left gaze and worse with head tilted right. What is the likely diagnosis and what should you do?

> *Right superior oblique palsy (possibly congenital).*

> The three-step test is consistent with a right superior oblique palsy, which is the most common (and therefore most likely) cause of long-standing vertical strabismus. But could there be some optical consideration behind the decompensation? You must check the old glasses, which may have had ground-in prism that you were not aware of, so that she became symptomatic when the new glasses were made without prism. There could also be accidental prism power due to displacement of the optical centers, due either to a manufacturing error or tilting of the frames. Of course, her control of the long-standing deviation may have also just deteriorated with time, so new prism glasses or strabismus surgery might be required to treat the double vision.

8. Your second-to-last appointment of the day is a 30-year-old new patient with "blurry vision." She cannot be refracted to better than 20/50 in either eye. Before commencing with pupil dilation and a medical evaluation for vision loss, what steps can you take to confirm that this is not a refractive problem?

> First, recheck visual acuity through the pinhole *with your best refraction in place*. If the visual acuity improves, there is still a refractive problem contributing to subnormal vision. Try using a higher-powered, handheld Jackson cross cylinder to refine the subjective refraction. At 20/50, the patient may not have good enough vision to detect a change in sharpness when you flip the ±0.25 D Jackson cross cylinder that is built into the phoropter. If the higher-powered Jackson cross cylinder does not help, look for irregular astigmatism in the retinoscopic reflex. If this is present, a hard contact lens overrefraction could improve corrected visual acuity. If visual acuity does not change with the pinhole, there are a few simple things to consider. Make sure that the eye chart in the room is properly calibrated and properly illuminated. Check visual acuity with both eyes open in case latent nystagmus is present. If vision does not improve with any of these measures, then she probably has a medical problem, and you will have to read a different book.

9. You are about to leave for the day, just in time to make your child's piano recital, when your last patient, a 39-year-old man, arrives 14 minutes late (just inside the grace period for cancellation) complaining of headaches and vaguely (yet with excruciating detail) describing recent "trouble" with his eyes: fatigue when reading, hard to focus but not blurry, "things like that." He has had to cut back on work

hours as a result of his discomfort. He has had the same glasses for many years. What issues should you consider when evaluating his headaches and asthenopia?

Asthenopia (eye strain) is a very common reason for dissatisfied patients. Recheck the refraction, as overcorrected myopia and latent hyperopia are common causes of eye strain. Cycloplegic refraction may be indicated in a case like this to detect more subtle latent hyperopia, especially in the prepresbyopic years, where the patient may have lost accommodative amplitude but developed an ability to dial in high amounts of their residual accommodation. It is useful to perform cover testing to look for a phoria or tropia. Finally, look for structural causes that may be contributing, such as dry eye, blepharitis, or early cataract.

10. **Your uncle-in-law, a retired ophthalmologist-engineer-surfer, is waiting for you as you try to exit the office. He wears glasses with lenses that incorporate rare earth metals and can only be made by a Shaolin Monk in the Henan province of China. The right lens has slab-off prism and a flat-top bifocal. The left lens is designed to be used with a contact lens to reduce aniseikonia due to his aphakic left eye and has a round-top bifocal. He has always had oblique astigmatism and he prefers to have the cylinder ground into the front of the lenses. He is no longer able to refract himself due to a recent surfing accident, and his glasses were badly scratched and the frames slightly bent in that same incident. He has also had asthenopia and mild blurring of vision since the accident, and the left contact lens does not feel right. He says that he trusts that your mastery of optics, refraction, and contact lenses to give him the perfect glasses and treat all of his symptoms. He adds that his niece, your wife, promised that you could fit him in for a visit tonight. (You know this is impossible because she has texted you 15 times in the last 9 minutes asking when you are going to arrive at the recital). What should you do?**

You have made it to the end of this book, so we know that you can handle all of his concerns and still make it to the recital on time. If not, pretend like you have never met the man, or do whatever is necessary to leave the clinic immediately. You need to make that recital. (Author's note: It would not be wise to refer him to any of this book's coauthors. We will look for you, we will find you, and we will punish you. And also thank you for buying this book. Or at least for reading it. And congratulations for making it to the end – probably at the last-minute before your exam!)

CHAPTER 20

Summary of Important Optics Formulas

If you only have time to look at one chapter in this book, here (Fig. 20.1) you will find the most important formulas in clinical optics, with details for each formula provided below.

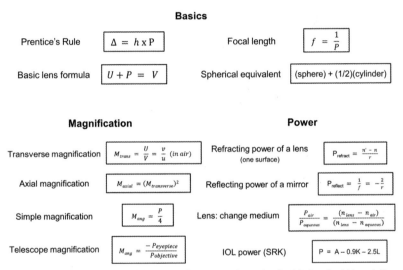

The Great Wall of Optics

Basics

Prentice's Rule $\quad \Delta = h \times P$

Focal length $\quad f = \dfrac{1}{P}$

Basic lens formula $\quad U + P = V$

Spherical equivalent $\quad$ (sphere) + (1/2)(cylinder)

Magnification

Transverse magnification $\quad M_{trans} = \dfrac{U}{V} = \dfrac{v}{u}$ (in air)

Axial magnification $\quad M_{axial} = (M_{transverse})^2$

Simple magnification $\quad M_{ang} = \dfrac{P}{4}$

Telescope magnification $\quad M_{ang} = \dfrac{-P_{eyepiece}}{P_{objective}}$

Power

Refracting power of a lens (one surface) $\quad P_{refract} = \dfrac{n' - n}{r}$

Reflecting power of a mirror $\quad P_{reflect} = \dfrac{1}{f} = -\dfrac{2}{r}$

Lens: change medium $\quad \dfrac{P_{air}}{P_{aqueous}} = \dfrac{(n_{lens} - n_{air})}{(n_{lens} - n_{aqueous})}$

IOL power (SRK) $\quad P = A - 0.9K - 2.5L$

Fig. 20.1 Handy reference to all of the most important formulas in this book. Abbreviations decoded below.

Basic Formulas

FOCAL LENGTH

$$f = \frac{1}{P}$$

f = focal length (meters)
P = lens power (diopters)

BASIC LENS EQUATION

$$U + P = V$$

U = vergence of rays entering lens (object rays)
P = vergence added by lens or mirror (power)
V = vergence of rays leaving lens (image rays)

PRENTICE'S RULE

$$\Delta = h \times P$$

Δ = induced prism (prism diopters)
h = distance from optical center (cm)
P = lens power (diopters)

SPHERICAL EQUIVALENT

$$SE = Sphere + \frac{1}{2} Cylinder$$

SE = spherical equivalent (diopters)
Sphere (diopters)
Cylinder (diopters)

CONVERT PLUS CYLINDER ↔ MINUS CYLINDER

1. New sphere = old sphere + old cylinder

2. New cylinder = same as old cylinder but opposite sign

3. New axis = change old axis by 90 degrees

Magnification

RETINAL IMAGE HEIGHT (OR OBJECT HEIGHT OF RETINAL IMAGE AT DISTANCE)

$$\frac{\text{object height}}{\text{retinal image height}} = \frac{\text{distance from nodal point}}{17 \text{ mm}}$$

SPECTACLE LENS MAGNIFICATION

$$Mag_{\text{spectacle lens}} = 2\% \text{ per diopter of power}$$

(Assume 12 mm vertex distance.)

TRANSVERSE MAGNIFICATION

$$Mag_{\text{transverse}} = \frac{\text{image height}}{\text{object height}} = \frac{U \text{ (object vergence)}}{V \text{ (image vergence)}} = \frac{v \text{ (image distance)}}{u \text{ (object distance)}}$$

AXIAL MAGNIFICATION

$$Mag_{\text{axial}} = \left(Mag_{\text{transverse}}\right)^2$$

SIMPLE MAGNIFIER

$$\text{Mag}_{\text{simple magnifier}} = \frac{P}{4} = P * 0.25 \text{ m}$$

D = lens power (diopters)
Standard reference distance = 1/4 m (0.25 m)
For nonstandard reference distance, replace 0.25 m with new reference distance

INDIRECT OPHTHALMOSCOPE LENS

$$\text{Mag}_{\text{transverse}} = \frac{P_{\text{eye}}}{P_{\text{lens}}} = \frac{60 \text{ D}}{P_{\text{lens}}}$$

TELESCOPE

$$\text{Mag}_{\text{telescope}} = -\frac{P_{\text{eyepiece}}}{P_{\text{objective}}}$$

Power Formulas

REFRACTING POWER OF A SPHERICAL SURFACE

$$P = \frac{n' - n}{r}$$

P = refracting power of surface (diopters)
(n′ − n) = difference in refractive index
r = radius of curvature of surface (meters)
To determine sign: use imaginary rectangle; color in the side with higher refractive
index

POWER OF A THIN LENS IMMERSED IN FLUID

$$\frac{P_{\text{air}}}{P_{\text{fluid}}} = \frac{(n_{\text{IOL}} - n_{\text{air}})}{(n_{\text{IOL}} - n_{\text{fluid}})}$$

P_{air} = power of lens in air
P_{fluid} = power of lens in fluid
n_{IOL} = refractive index of lens
n_{fluid} = refractive index of fluid
n_{air} = 1.00

REFLECTING POWER OF A SPHERICAL MIRROR

$$P_{\text{reflecting}} = \frac{1}{f} = -\frac{2}{r}$$

$P_{\text{reflecting}}$ = surface reflecting power (diopters)
f = focal length (meters)
r = radius of curvature (meter)

INTRAOCULAR LENS POWER (SRK FORMULA)

$$P_{IOL} = A - 2.5(L) - 0.9(K)$$

P_{IOL} = recommended power for emmetropia (diopters)
A = A constant
L = axial length (mm)
K = keratometry reading (diopters)
SRK = Sanders, Retzlaff, and Kraft

Table of Reciprocals

Commonly used reciprocals are highlighted in Table 20.1.

TABLE 20.1 ■ Simple Reciprocals
(Most Common in Bold)

1/1	1
1/2	0.50
1/3	0.33
1/4	0.25
1/5	0.20
1/6	0.17
1/7	0.14
1/8	0.125
1/9	0.11
1/10	0.10
1/11	0.09
1/12	0.083
1/20	0.05
1/25	0.04

INDEX

Note: Page numbers followed by '*f*' indicate figures, '*b*' indicate boxes, and '*t*' indicate tables.